Definitions, Protocols and Guidelines in Genetic Hearing Impairment

Definitions, Protocols and Guidelines in Genetic Hearing Impairment

Edited by

ALESSANDRO MARTINI MD, MANUELA MAZZOLI MD,
ANDREW READ PhD, DAFYDD STEPHENS FRCP

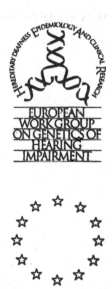

W
WHURR PUBLISHERS
LONDON AND PHILADELPHIA

© 2001 Whurr Publishers Ltd

First published 2001 by Whurr Publishers Ltd
19b Compton Terrace, London N1 2UN, England and
325 Chestnut Street, Philadelphia PA 19106, USA

British Library Cataloguing in Publication Data

A catalogue record for this book is available from the British Library.

ISBN 1 86156 188 1

Contents

Contributors

Eliza Calzolari
Institute of Medical Genetics, University of Ferrara, Ferrara, Italy

Cor Cremers
Department of Otorhinolaryngology, University of Nijmegen, Belgium

Adrian Davis
MRC Institute of Hearing Research, University Park, Nottingham, England

Frank Declau
Department of Otorhinolaryngology, University of Antwerp, Belgium

Francesca Gualandi
Institute of Medical Genetics, University of Ferrara, Ferrara, Italy

Stavros Hatzopoulos
Audiology – ENT, University of Ferrara, Ferrara, Italy

Patrick Huygen
Department of Otolaryngology, University Hospital, Nijmegen, Netherlands

Howard Jacobs
Department of Genetics, University of Tampere, Tampere, Finland

Veronica Kennedy
Welsh Hearing Institute, University Hospital of Wales, Cardiff, Wales

Geneviève Lina-Granade
Department of Audiology, Hôpital Edward Herriot, Lyon, France

Linda Luxon
Department of Audiological Medicine, Institute of Child Health, London, England

Alessandro Martini
Audiology – ENT, University of Ferrara, Ferrara, Italy

Manuela Mazzoli
Audiology – ENT, University of Ferrara, Ferrara, Italy

Claes Möller
Department of Audiology, Salgrenska Hospital, Göteborg, Sweden

Robert Mueller
Department of Medical Genetics, University of Leeds, England

Valerie Newton
Department of Audiology, University of Manchester, Manchester, England

Lars Ödkvist
Department of Otolaryngology, University Hospital, Linköping, Sweden

Eva Orzan
Department of Audiology, University of Padua, Padua, Italy

Agnete Parving
Department of Audiology, Bispebjerg Hospital, Copenhagen, Denmark

Andrew Read
Department of Medical Genetics, St Mary's Hospital, Manchester, England

Alberto Sensi
Institute of Medical Genetics, University of Ferrara, Ferrara, Italy

Richard Smith
Department of Otolaryngology, University of Iowa, Iowa City, Iowa, USA

Dafydd Stephens
Welsh Hearing Institute, University Hospital of Wales, Cardiff, Wales

Guy Van Camp
Department of Medical Genetics, University of Antwerp, Antwerp, Belgium

Paul Van de Heyning
Department of Otorhinolaryngology, University of Antwerp, Belgium

Floris Wuyts
Department of Otolaryngology, University Hospital, Antwerp, Belgium

Fei Zhao
Welsh Hearing Institute, University Hospital of Wales, Cardiff, Wales

Chapter 1
Introduction: putting together the pieces of the auditory puzzle

ALESSANDRO MARTINI, MANUELA MAZZOLI, ANDREW READ, DAFYDD STEPHENS

Cracking the code

Cor Cremers started his *lectio professoralis* by going directly to the core of what has been most significant in the field of audiology in recent years: the discovery that many genes cause deafness and thus the beginning of an understanding of the normal and defective auditory codes. The import-ance of this event for the scientific community is confirmed by the appear-ance in *The New England Journal of Medicine* of the editorial 'A new era in the genetics of deafness' by Karen Steel.

One in every 1,000 new-born babies suffers from congenital severe or profound hearing impairment. Moreover, epidemiological studies show that the percentages of the population having a hearing impairment exceeding 45 dB HL and 65 dB HL are respectively about 1.3% and 0.3% between the ages of 30 and 50 years, and 7.4% and 2.3% between the ages of 60 and 70 years (Davis, 1989).

Loss of hearing has long been considered a permanent effect conse-quent on such factors as infections, ototoxicity, trauma and ageing. In recent years, molecular biology and molecular genetics have made a major contribution to the understanding of the normal and defective inner ear, not only in congenital profound hearing impairment but also in late-onset/progressive hearing impairment.

Although many families with autosomal dominant (AD) progressive hereditary hearing impairment have been reported in the literature, no epidemiological information exists on the prevalence of genetic hearing impairment in the adult population (Parving, 1996). The majority of these adult-onset forms result from an interaction of environmental and genetic

1

factors (Sill et al., 1994). Animal studies have provided valuable information on the degenerative processes developing in the auditory system as a function of age (Steel, 1991) and a number of syndromes are recognized both in the human and in the mouse, in which hearing loss presents with a late onset (Brown and Steel, 1996). In the 'neuroepithelial defects' group, the primary defect lies in the neuroepithelia of the inner ear: the hair cells ultimately degenerate, but some developmental defects can be detected long before the onset of degeneration (Steel, 1996). Genetically determined hearing impairment may develop at any age either as the sole manifestation of the mutant gene, as part of an inherited syndrome, or as interaction with exogenous factors (Parving, 1996). In fact, it is possible that mutations in some genes render the ear more susceptible to environmental factors causing inner ear damage (noise exposure, infection, injury and ototoxic drugs) (Van Camp, Coucke and Willems, 1996).

The HEAR project

In September 1994, when a Preparatory Workshop for the Constitution of a European study group on genetic deafness was held in Milan, only four loci of non syndromal hearing impairment and only three genes responsible for syndromal hearing impairment had been discovered.

After approval from the Commission of the European Community, during the years 1996–9, the group of researchers known as the European Concerted Action HEAR (Hereditary Deafness: Epidemiology and Clinical Research) organized scientific meetings[1] and produced documents[2] with the aim of co-ordinating research on the genetics of hearing impairment.

This project stimulated a considerable amount of work in this field leading to developments in molecular genetics and the mapping of human loci associated with hearing disorders (Figures 1 and 2). The numerous and scattered loci mapped reflect a heterogeneous set of genes and mechanisms responsible for human hearing and suggest a complicated interaction between these genes (Lalwani and Castelein, 1999).

The importance of establishing common terminology and definitions and of co-ordinating the multidisciplinary approach was stressed during the preparatory meeting in Milan. The idea was to deal with the problem of combining clinical in-depth family and phenotypic studies with basic molecular genetic and gene mapping methods in a more standardized way, with the aim of establishing stable international collaboration. The idea was also to create a bank of updated information on these disorders that would be useful not only to experts but to the entire scientific community in identifying sources of information and specialized centres to which specific cases may be referred.

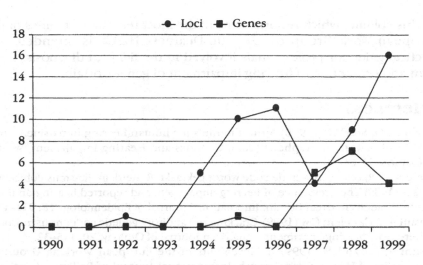

Figure 1.1: Non-syndromal hearing impairment – new loci and genes identified by year.

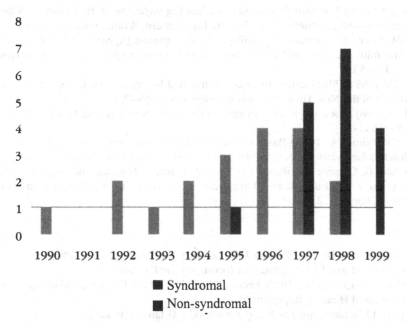

Figure 1.2: New syndromal and non-syndromal hearing impairment genes identified by year. The genes underlying most syndromes have now been identified, hence the fall in the rate of identification since 1997.

The clinical expression of different conditions (autosomal dominant, autosomal recessive, X-linked) was investigated in an attempt to find clues suggesting the underlying genetic condition (see Chapters 14 to 17).

This volume, which reports some of the most relevant outcomes of the European Work Group on Genetic Deafness HEAR, is intended as a practical guide for professionals involved in the fields of diagnosis, treatment and prevention of hearing impairment of genetic origin.

References

Brown SDM, Steel KP (1996) Mouse models for human hearing impairment. In A Martini, A Read, D Stephens (eds), Genetics and Hearing Impairment, Whurr, London, 53–63.

Cremers CWRJ (1998) Horen de code wordt gekraakt. Rotterdam: Erasmus Publishing.

Davis A (1989) The prevalence of hearing impairment and reported hearing disability among adults in Great Britain. International Journal of Epidemiology 18: 911–17.

Lalwani A K, Castelein CM (1999) Cracking the auditory genetic code: nonsyndromic hereditary hearing imprimente. American Journal of Otology, 20: 115–32.

Martini A, Mazzoli M (1999) Achievements of the European Working Group on Genetics of Hearing Imprimente. International Journal of Pediatric Otorhinolaryngology, 49: S155–S158.

Parving A (1996) Epidemiology of genetic hearing impairment. In A Martini, A Read, D Stephens (eds), Genetics and Hearing Impairment, Whurr, London, 73–81.

Sill AM, Stick MJ, Prenger VL, Phillips SL, Boughman JA, Arnos KS (1994) Genetic epidemiologic study of hearing impairment. American Journal of Human Genetics 54: 149–53.

Steel KP (1991) Similarities between mice and humans with hereditary deafness. Annals of the New York Academy of Science 630: 68–79.

Steel K (1998) A new era in the genetics of deafness. New England Journal of Medicine 339: 1545–7.

Steel KP, Palmer A (1996) Basic mechanisms of hearing impairment. In A Martini, A Read, D Stephens (eds), Genetics and Hearing Impairment, Whurr, London, 73–81.

van Camp G, Coucke P, Willems PJ (1996) Autosomal dominant non-syndromal hearing loss. A Martini, A Read, D Stephens (eds), Genetics and Hearing Impairment, Whurr, London, 213–20

Notes

1. Copenhagen, 16–18 February 1996, groups 1-2 (promoted by A Parving).
   London, 11 April 1996, group 4a (promoted by E Calzolari).
   Milan, 11–13 October 1996, Second Workshop of the European Working Group on Genetics of Hearing Impairment,
   Lyon, 17 January, groups 1–2 (promoted by G Lina-Granade).
   Athens, 16 November 1996, joint meetings of European projects AHEAD-HEAR-PAN.
   Genova, 19 May 1997, group 5 (promoted by A Read).
   Aalborg, 26 May 1997, group 3 (promoted by L Luxon and C Moeller).
   Prague 18 June 1997, joint meetings of European projects AHEAD-HEAR-PAN.
   Bethesda, August 1997, group 5 (promoted by A Read).
   Ferrara, 10–12 October 1997, groups 1-2-3 (promoted by D Stephens, A Parving and A Martini).

Anversa, February 1999, group 4b (promoted by P van de Heyning).

Bibione, 4–7 March 1999, Third International Meeting of the European Working Group on Genetics of Hearing Impairment.

2. Martini A, Stephens D, Read A (1996) Genetics and Hearing Impairment. London: Whurr.

Stephens D, Read A, Martini A (1998) Development in Genetic Hearing impairment. London: Whurr.

Martini A, Mazzoli M (1999) Achievements of the European Working Group on Genetics of Hearing Impairment. Int J Ped Otorynolaringol 49: S155–S158.

Read A, Stephens D, Martini A (eds) (1999) Br J Audiol 33: 5.

HEAR Infoletter 1–6.

Hereditary Hearing Loss Homepage (sponsored) (http://www.via.ac.be/dnalab/hhh).

HEAR Homepage (http://hear.unife.it).

Part I
Terminology and
definitions

Chapter 2
Audiological terms

DAFYDD STEPHENS

The aim of this chapter is to provide precise, acceptable and current definitions of various audiological terms currently used in the context of genetic hearing impairment. There exists much confusion, even among audiologists, as to the most appropriate terms to be used and, within this section, the most relevant terms were adopted following considerable discussion. Study group 1 of the Concerted Action programme undertook this work and the active participants are listed at the end of the chapter.

We strongly recommend the universal use of these terms by all those working in the field of genetic hearing impairment and, indeed, with all aspects of hearing impairment.

Within this section we shall begin with the broad definitions of disablements, followed by the more specific audiometric measures and finally define the different types of impairment related to lesions in the various parts of the auditory system.

Disablements/disabilities (after WHO, 1980; 1997; 1999; Stephens and Hétu, 1991).

'Disablements' was the collective term introduced in the World Health Organization classification of impairments, disabilities and handicaps (WHO, 1980), which brought together a unified terminology that could be applied to the effects of all kinds of disorders ranging from audition to locomotion. In the latest amendment it is confusingly replaced by the old term 'disabilities'.

Through the 1980s and 1990s a number of weaknesses in the original classification were highlighted and extensions of the classification were described. A new classification (ICIDH – 2), introduced as a draft in 1997 (WHO, 1997), set out to incorporate many of these proposals, which have

9

been amended in the Beta-2 draft published in 1999 (WHO, 1999). While it still has a number of shortcomings in detail, it represents a major advance, which should be useful to those working in this field.

The new classification aims to move away from the negative terms of 'impairment', 'disability' and 'handicap' and replace them with the neutral terms of 'body function and structure', 'activity' and 'participation'.

Activity – is the performance of a task or action by an individual.

Activity limitations – (formerly 'disabilities') are difficulties an individual may have in the performance of activities.

Body functions – are the physiological or psychological functions of body systems.

Body structures – are anatomical parts of the body such as the auricle or tympanic membrane.

Disablement (now disability) – An umbrella term covering the negative dimensions of impairments, activity, limitations and participation restrictions (formerly referred to as disabilities and handicaps). The relationship between these is shown in Figure 2.1.

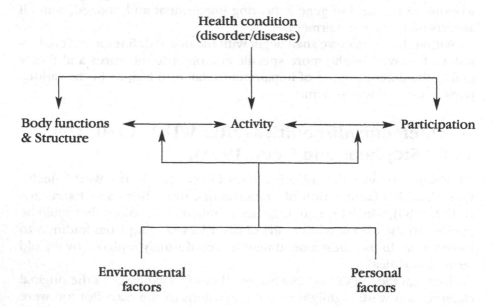

Figure 2.1: Relationship between impairments, activity limitations and participation restrictions.

Impairments – Problems in body function or structure as a significant deviation or loss.

Participation – An individual's involvement in life situations.

Participation restrictions – Formerly called 'handicaps', these are problems that an individual may have in the manner or extent of involvement in life situations.

Tinnitus – The conscious experience of a sound that originates in an involuntary manner in the head of its owner or may appear to him or her to do so (Coles, 1997). (Short-duration tinnitus after noise exposure and bursts of tinnitus lasting less than five minutes are normally excluded from this definition.) In ICIDH-2 (WHO, 1999) it is regarded as an impairment analogous to vertigo.

The terms 'hearing disability' and 'handicap', or even 'hearing handicap' are often loosely applied to hearing impaired people. These terms are not usually relevant to studies on genetic hearing impairment and *should be avoided*. Indeed, in the revised World Health Organization definition of disablements (1999) they have been replaced, with some changes, by the terms 'activity limitation' and 'participation restriction'.

Audiometric measures

The following classification is based on the earlier approaches of Parving and Newton (1995) and of Liu and Xu (1994) with some modifications following the experience of using those systems.

Audiometric configurations

Deafness – This term has many different meanings in different contexts and *should be avoided* in the context of genetic hearing impairment. Equally the term *hearing loss* is inappropriate in that in many genetic disorders involving the auditory system, normal function has never been present and so has not been lost. *Hearing impairment* is the term of choice.

Hearing threshold level – The level of hearing of the individual for pure tones compared with internationally agreed standards (ISO 389, 1991).

Hearing threshold levels – Applied to the better hearing ear, averaged across 500, 1,000, 2,000 and 4,000 Hz. If these verbal descriptors are used, the actual hearing level should also be included.

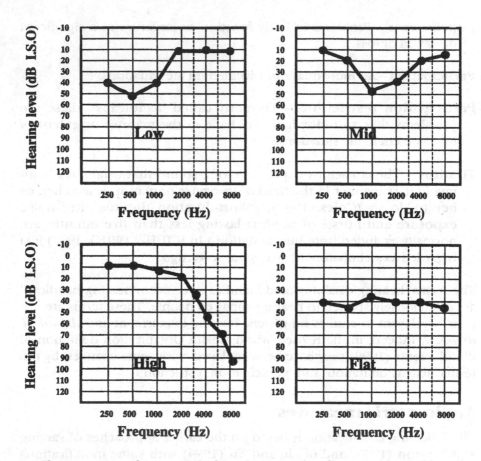

Low frequency ascending – >15 dB from the poorer low frequency thresholds to the higher frequencies.

Mid-frequency U-shaped – >15 dB difference between the poorest thresholds in the mid-frequencies, and those at higher and lower frequencies.

High frequency

    Gently sloping – 15–29 dB difference between the mean of 500 and 1,000 Hz and the mean of 4,000 and 8,000 Hz.

    Steeply sloping – >30 dB difference between the above frequencies.

Flat – <15 dB difference between the mean of 250/500 Hz thresholds, the mean of 1 and 2 kHz and the mean of 4 and 8 kHz.

Figure 2.2: Audiometric configurations.

Mild – over 20 dB and less than 40 dB

Moderate – over 40 dB and less than 70 dB

Severe – over 70 dB and less than 95 dB

Profound – equal to and over 95 dB

Frequency ranges

Low – Up to and equal to 500 Hz
Mid – Over 500 Hz up to and equal to 2,000 Hz
High – Over 2,000 Hz up to and equal to 8,000 Hz
Extended high – Over 8,000 Hz

Types of hearing impairment

This final section provides working definitions of the specific types of hearing impairment arising from pathology in different parts of the auditory pathway. It is likely that in the future with better understanding of specific lesions within the cochlea (for example, outer hair cell versus stria vascularis) subdivisions of 'sensory' will be developed.

Asymmetrical hearing impairment – >10 dB difference between the ears in at least two frequencies, with the pure tone average in the better ear worse than 20 dB HL.

Central – A sensorineural hearing loss related to a disease or deformity of the central nervous system rostral to the cochlear nerve.

Conductive – Related to disease or deformity of the outer/middle ears. Audiometrically there are normal bone conduction thresholds (<20 dB) and an air–bone gap >15 dB averaged over 0.5, 1 and 2 kHz.

Mixed – Related to combined involvement of the outer/middle ears and the inner ear/cochlear nerve. Audiometrically >20 dB HL in the bone conduction threshold together with >15 dB air–bone gap averaged over 0.5, 1 and 2 kHz.

Neural – A subdivision of sensorineural related to a disease or deformity in the cochlear nerve.

Progressive hearing impairment – A deterioration of >15 dB in the pure tone average within a 10-year period. Results in those aged over 50 years should be treated with some caution. In all cases, the time-scale and patient age should be specified.

Sensorineural – Related to disease/deformity of the inner ear/cochlear nerve with an air/bone gap <15 dB averaged over 0.5, 1 and 2 kHz.

Sensory – A subdivision of sensorineural related to a disease or deformity in the cochlea.

Unilateral hearing impairment – One ear only has either >20 dB pure tone average or one frequency exceeding 50 dB, with the other ear better than or equal to 20 dB.

Acknowledgements

The following members of study group 1 provided vital active participation in the development of Chapters 1, 7, 8 and 9: Geneviève Lina-Granade, Stavros Hatzopoulos, Alessandro Martini, Manuela Mazzoli, Valerie Newton, Eva Orzan, David Parker, Martti Sorri, Kunigunde Weltzl-Möller and Fei Zhao.

We are grateful to Stig Arlinger for drawing our attention to discrepancies with ISO definitions which have subsequently been amended.

References

Coles RRA (1997) Tinnitus. In Stephens D (ed.) Scott-Brown's Otolaryngology. 6 edn. Volume 2. Oxford: Butterworth-Heinemann.
Davis A (1995) Hearing in Adults. London: Whurr.
Liu X and Xu L (1994) Non syndromic hearing loss. An analysis of audiograms. Annals of Otology, Rhinology and Laryngology 103: 428-33.
Parving A, Newton V (1995) Guidelines for description of inherited hearing loss. Journal of Audiological Medicine 4, ii–iii.
Stephens D, Francis M (1996) The detection of carriers of genetic hearing loss. In Martini A, Read A, Stephens D (eds) Genetic and Hearing Impairment. London: Whurr, pp 100–8.
Stephens D, Hétu R (1991) Impairment, disability and handicap in audiology: towards a consensus. Audiology 30: 185–200.
World Health Organization (1980) International Classification of Impairments, Disabilities and Handicaps. Geneva: World Health Organization.
World Health Organization (1997) ICIDH-2: International Classification of Impairments, Activities and Participation. Geneva: World Health Organization.
World Health Organization (1999) ICIDH-2: International Classification of Functioning and Disability. Beta-2 draft, full version. Geneva: World Health Organization. (Website http://www.who.ch/icidh.)

Chapter 3
Vestibular terms

Claes Möller

The inner ear consists of two parts with close anatomical, physiological and functional resemblance, so a diagnosis of genetic or non-genetic hearing impairment should include a vestibular assessment.

This would help to classify and differentiate between hearing disorders, reveal genetic vestibular disorders and give a prognosis of possible progression. Vestibular assessment would also help patients to understand possible symptoms of clumsiness and thus encourage them to compensate for a vestibular deficiency by physical activity.

It is our hope that the vestibular test protocol will be used in order to simplify evaluation and to standardize vestibular assessment.

Asymmetry – The percentage difference between the peak slow eye velocities to the right and the left.

Ataxia – Usually means unsteadiness. The definition does not state where the lesion is localized. The term vestibulo-cerebellar ataxia usually implies a central nervous lesion.

Caloric testing – The test can be performed in many ways. The most common procedures are bithermal-binaural (30°C and 44°C) water applied to the external ear canal. The test results show hypoactivity, hyperactivity, asymmetry or absent responses. Ice water calorics (8°C) are used to confirm areflexia or total canal paresis.

Canal paresis – Means that there is no nystagmus as a response to caloric irrigation. This suggests that the vestibular apparatus does not work.

Dizziness – This encompasses any discomfort other than pain, related to the head, and is not a useful term in the context of genetic hearing impairment.

Electro-oculography (nystagmography) – A method of recording nystagmus by using electrodes placed at the outer canthus and the forehead.

Fistula test – A nystagmus that appears when negative or positive pressure is applied to the ear canal.

Lightheadedness – A feeling of 'going to faint' or 'things turning dark' without actual loss of consciousness. This is also of little use in the context of genetic hearing impairment.

Nyst agmus – A biphasic oscillation of the eyes initiated by an imbalance of the eye position resulting in a drift of the eyes (slow phase) and a corrective movement (fast phase). Nystagmus can be separated into:

- *Spontaneous nystagmus* – nystagmus present, usually without fixation (in darkness). The direction can be horizontal, vertical or torsional. The fast phase of the eye movement is the direction of the nystagmus.
- *Gaze-evoked nystagmus* – a nystagmus that appears when looking 30° to the left or right.
- *Positional nystagmus* – a nystagmus that appears in different head positions.
- *Head-shaking nystagmus* – a nystagmus elicited by head shaking, usually 10 times. A persistent nystagmus after head shaking is patho-logical.

Saccadic eye movements – Fast eye movements directing the gaze to a point of fixation. The saccades can be both voluntary and involuntary.

Smooth pursuit eye movements – A slow eye movement that enables clear fixation of a moving object by keeping it on the fovea.

Unsteadiness – Loss of equilibrium in relation to the environment. It is often described by the patient as 'bumping into things' or 'losing the footing'.

Velocity – The velocity of the eye movement is the mathematical derivative of the sine wave curve for displacement. The velocity of a nystagmus is usually measured as the velocity of the slow phase eye movement (degree/s).

Vertigo – An actual sensation of motion in which either the patient or the environment moves. The movement is often rotatory.

Vestibular-ocular reflex (VOR) – A head movement will cause endolymph flow in the semicircular canals. The excitation and inhibition due to cupular movement will cause an eye movement opposite to the head movement.

Video-oculography – A method for recording eye movements using a video technique.

Chapter 4
Epidemiological terms

ADRIAN DAVIS

The aim of this chapter is to provide background definitions of the main terms used in the epidemiology of genetic hearing impairment. They are general epidemiological terms equally applied to all types of disorder.

Cohort – the component of the population that is born during a particular period and identified by period of birth, so that its characteristics (for example, prevalence of childhood hearing impairment, age at first hearing aid fitting) can be ascertained as it enters successive time and age periods.

Cohort study – has now come to mean many things such as follow-up study, prospective study, or longitudinal study. A cohort study is essential to understanding change over time and the impact of services for hearing-impaired children. (A study of cases arriving at a clinic, for example, in the year 1996 is not adequate for giving an unbiased estimate of the effect of service provision.)

Incidence – the number of new instances of a specific condition (such as hearing impairment from meningitis) occurring during a certain period in a specified population.

Incidence rate – is the rate at which this occurs per standard population – for example 10 new cases per year per 100,000 children.

Odds ratio – (sometimes known as 'relative odds'). The ratio of two odds. The term 'odds' is defined differently, depending on what is under discussion. Consider the following concerning distribution of disease given exposure to a risk:

	Exposed	Not exposed
Disease	a	b
No disease	c	d

where a . . . d are the numbers of people in each category, then the odds ratio is $(a \times d)/(b \times c)$.

The exposure odds ratio for a set of case control data is the ratio of the odds in favour of exposure among the cases (a/b) to the odds in favour of exposure among the non-cases $(c/d) \geq (a \times d)/(b \times c)$. For a rare disease (<2% prevalence of incidence) this is a good estimate of the risk ratio.

Odds score – is synonymous with odds ratio.

Population study – the whole collection of units from which a sample may be drawn; not necessarily a population of people – it may be a collection of hearing aid clinics, schools for the deaf, and so forth. The sample is intended to give results that are representative of the population as a whole. Thus when attempting a prevalence study, if there are n children with hearing impairment in the study, and the whole population of children is N, then the prevalence rate is $(n \times 100/N)\%$. In this case we must be sure that the n hearing impaired children really come from all the birth cohorts of children represented by the population of N, and that there is co-terminosity of n and N in terms of geographical boundaries. It is quite common to either underestimate n (because not all children with a given condition have been found) or to confuse populations, for example because of migration of children into or out of particular districts. A population study is one in which the sample is carefully selected for representativeness of the whole population.

Positive predictive value (PPV) – The proportion of those who fail a screening test who have a specified condition.

Prevalence – The total number of instances of a specified condition (for example, Pendred syndrome) in a given population at a specific time.

Prevalence rate – The number who have the condition or attribute divided by the population at risk at a point in time (or midway through a period).

Risk – The probability that an event will occur; for example, that a child will have a hearing impairment of 50 dB HL or greater.

Risk ratio – The ratio of two risks, for example, the ratio of the probability that a child will be hearing impaired if there are two brothers with congenital hearing impairment to that of being hearing impaired if no relatives are congenitally hearing impaired.

Risk odds ratio – The ratio of the odds in favour of getting a disease if exposed, to the odds in favour of getting the disease if not exposed. The odds derived from a cohort study are an estimate of this.

Sensitivity – The proportion of target individuals (for example, truly hearing impaired) in the screened population who are correctly identified by the screening test = true positive rate. (Screen sensitivity has to be distinguished from programme sensitivity, which is screen sensitivity multiplied by the coverage of the programme.)

Specificity – The proportion of truly non-target (for example normally hearing) people who are correctly identified by the screening test = true negative rate.

Yield – the number or proportion of cases of a specified condition accurately identified.

Chapter 5
Genetic terms

ANDREW READ

Allele – One or several possible forms of a particular gene, which may or may not be pathological.

Allelic heterogeneity – Allelic heterogeneity is seen when many different mutations at the same genetic locus can cause a disease. This is almost always the case – for example Waardenburg syndrome Type 1 is always caused by mutations at the *PAX3* locus, but different families usually have different *PAX3* mutations.

Association – co-occurrence at a frequency significantly different from statistical chance. Characters may be associated in a phenotype, or a genetic condition may be associated in population with a particular allele at a locus. Associations can be positive or negative.

Autosomal inheritance – The transmission of an allele carried on an autosome. Autosomal inheritance is suspected when a character can be transmitted by a parent of either sex to a child of either sex.

Autosomal dominant – The pedigree pattern seen when an allele at an autosomal locus causes a dominant character.

Autosome – A chromosome other than a sex chromosome (X or Y).

Pedigree description of autosomal dominant inheritance. Both males and females can be affected. The disorder is transmitted from generation to generation and can be transmitted in all possible ways: female to female, female to male, male to female and male to male (this latter specifically distinguishes autosomal from X-linked inheritance). Formal segregation studies to show that the ratio is 1:1 affected:non-affected in individual families is not usually possible. In small families the mode of inheritance can be difficult to determine, but transmission of a rare condition across three generations is good evidence for dominant inheritance. Many dominant conditions are variable (even within families) and may skip generations.

Autosomal recessive – The pedigree pattern seen when an allele at an autosomal locus causes a recessive character.

Pedigree description of autosomal recessive inheritance. Both males and females can be affected. If the parents of affected individual(s) are consanguineous, then recessive inheritance is more likely, but not certain. Usually only individuals within one sibship are affected; parents and other relatives are usually unaffected. In most cases there is only one affected individual in the family, making the pedigree pattern hard to identify as autosomal recessive, but in large multiply inbred kindreds, affected individuals may be seen in several branches of the family.

Carrier – An unaffected person with one pathogenic and one normal allele at a locus. Best restricted to heterozygotes for recessive conditions, but the word is sometimes applied to unaffected people with a gene for an incompletely penetrant or late-onset dominant condition.

Cousin – In genetics, the word 'cousin' should be used only as part of the specific terms 'first cousin', 'second cousin' and so forth, and not as a general term for 'relative'. *First cousins* are the offspring of sibs. Two people are *second cousins* if their parents are first cousins.

Degree of relationship – *First-degree relatives* are parents, offspring, sibs; these relatives share half their genes. *Second-degree relatives* are grandparents, grandchildren, uncles, aunts, nephews, nieces, half-sibs; these relatives share one quarter of their genes. *Third-degree relatives* share one eighth of their genes; first cousins are the main category ascertained in practice.

Dominant – A character that is manifest when present in the heterozygous state.

Familial – Tending to run in families (for genetic or other reasons).

Genotype – The genetic constitution of a person. One can talk of the genotype at a single locus, or the overall genotype. (Cf. **phenotype**.)

Haplotype – A series of alleles at linked loci on the same physical chromosome.

Hereditary – Transmitted in a family by genetic means.

Heterozygous – Having two different alleles at a locus.

Homozygous – Having two identical alleles at a locus.

Inbred – A person is inbred whose parents are blood relatives (consanguineous). Since ultimately everybody is related, a practical working definition is that the parents are second cousins or closer relatives.

Kindred – An extended family.

Locus – The position that a gene occupies on a chromosome. People have a pair of each autosome, so a person has two alleles (identical or different) at each autosomal locus.

Locus heterogeneity – Locus heterogeneity is seen when indistinguishable Mendelian disorders can be caused by mutations at more than one locus. This is a common finding in genetics; for example, Usher syndrome Type 1 can be caused by mutations at loci on the long arm of chromosome 14 (14q31), the long arm of chromosome 11 (11q13), the short arm of chromosome 11 (11p13) or at least three other loci.

Lod score – The statistical outcome of linkage analysis. The logarithm of the odds of linkage versus no linkage. A lod score above +3 gives significant evidence for linkage, and a score below −2 gives significant evidence against linkage.

Mitochondrial inheritance – Each mitochondrion contains several copies of a small circular DNA molecule containing 37 genes concerned with mitochondrial function. Mitochondria are transmitted in the egg but not in the sperm. When a condition is caused by a mutation in the mitochondrial genome, mothers pass it on to their children of both sexes, but fathers do not transmit it. Pathological mutations usually affect only a proportion of the mitochondria (heteroplasmy), and the consequences of inheriting a mitochondrial mutation can be very variable, both between individuals in a family and between different tissues in the same individual. Characteristically, mitochondrial disease affects more than one organ system – for example hearing impairment and diabetes.

Non-penetrance – Describes the situation when a person carrying a gene for a dominant character does not manifest the character. This is because of the effects of other genes or of environmental factors.

Nuclear family – Parents and their children; any larger family can be called a kindred.

Obligate carrier – A person who is necessarily a carrier by virtue of the pedigree structure. For autosomal recessive conditions, this normally means the parents of an affected person; for X-linked recessive conditions, it normally means a woman who has affected or carrier offspring and also affected brothers or maternal uncles. A woman who has only affected offspring is not an obligate carrier of an X-linked condition, because new mutations are frequent in X-linked (but not autosomal recessive) pedigrees.

Offspring – A person's offspring are his or her children, regardless of their age.

Penetrance – the probability that a phenotype will be seen with a given genotype.

Phenotype – the observed characteristics of a person (including the result of clinical examination). Compare with **genotype.**

Recessive – A character that is manifest only in the homozygous state, and not in heterozygotes.

Sibship – A set of sibs.

Sibs (siblings) – Brothers and sisters, regardless of sex.

Syndrome – The occurrence together of several features having a presumed common cause.

X-linked inheritance – X-linked inheritance is seen when a condition is caused by an allele located on the X chromosome.

Pedigree description of X-linked inheritance. Many X-linked diseases are seen only or almost only in males; where females are affected they may be more mildly or more variably affected. The X chromosome is transmitted to a male from his mother and never from his father, so male to male transmission rules out X-linked inheritance. The line of inheritance in a pedigree must go exclusively through females or affected males. All daughters of an affected male are carriers. The distinction between dominant and recessive is less clear-cut with X-linked than with autosomal conditions; however, female heterozygotes for most X-linked conditions are not obviously affected (even though testing may reveal sub-clinical signs of affection), so these conditions are X-linked recessive.

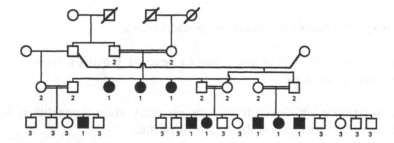

1. Typical autosomal dominant pedigree pattern, with priorities for sampling indicated. NB transmission by affected males rules out mitochondrial inheritance. * This person has an affected parent and an affected child, but is herself unaffected. This is an example of non-penetrance.

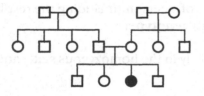

2. Typical autosomal recessive pedigree pattern, mimicking a sporadic condition. Such families are not useful for linkage studies, but may be useful for mutation detection.

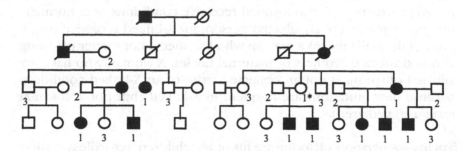

3. An example of a multiply-inbred pedigree with many cases of an autosomal recessive condition. Such rare families are exceptionally valuable for linkage analysis. Priorities for sampling are indicated.

Figure 5.1: Examples of pedigree patterns.

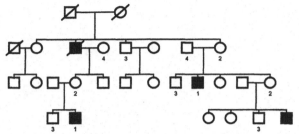

4. X-linked recessive pedigree pattern, showing likely priorities for sampling.

Figure 5.1: cont.

Part II
Protocols

Chapter 6
Audiometric investigation of probands

DAFYDD STEPHENS

Introduction

The aim of this chapter is to provide a set of recommendations as to the minimum basic battery of hearing tests that should be used in the assessment of the probands and other primarily affected individuals within a family. Other tests may be added according to the specific dysfunction involved and the policy of the department concerned. The tests listed below are all important in the definition of the specific phenotype.

Following a survey of participating centres throughout Europe and discussions with the project working group it was recommended that the following should comprise a minimum set for children aged over 5 years and for adults:

Acoustic reflex thresholds (ARTs) 500–4,000 Hz + WBN ipsilateral and contralateral, with non-acoustic reflexes if no responses are present with acoustical stimulation. The non-acoustic reflexes should be evoked by a puff of air in the eye.

Békésy audiometry (or rapid sweep audioscan) 125 Hz–8 kHz; 2.5 dB/s attenuation, 45 or 60 s/oct with a pulsed tone (interrupted) stimulus. This gives better information on the configuration of the audiogram, and should be performed in all cases with mild or moderate hearing impairment and old enough to perform the test. If Békésy audiometry is not available, pure tone audiometry should be performed including the half-octave intervals (0.75, 1.5, 3 and 6 kHz).

Bone conduction – Always masked – to be performed except when hearing is normal at the low frequencies.

29

Clinical tests – Voice, tuning fork, Barany box.

Oto-admittance 220–250 Hz probe tone, +200 to –400 daPa should be performed unless the tympanic membrane is perforated.

Pure tone audiogram – Air conduction (with masking where indicated) at least at octave frequencies 125 Hz–8 kHz.

The following test should be performed when clinically indicated:

Auditory brainstem response testing (ABR) – This should normally be performed on individuals with unilateral or asymmetrical hearing impairment or if there is a reason to suspect a neural or brainstem cause for the hearing impairment.

Children under five years of age

As many as possible of the tests recommended for over 5s should be included; transcient oto-acoustic emissions (TOAEs) testing and ABR should be performed when a full test battery is not possible. The other tests used will be age dependent but should include at least one test of low frequency threshold and one of high frequency threshold.

Progression

A full audiogram or Békésy audiometry should be performed after one year and subsequently at two-year intervals unless there are any significant changes in the hearing level. It provides a clearer picture of the stepwise progression of the hearing impairment that may occur in certain families.

Tinnitus

It should be noted whether or not this symptom is present.

Balance tests

These are defined by study group 3 in Chapter 9.

Other tests

The following are **not** in the minimum set. It is felt that in general they do not contribute significantly to the differentiation between different phenotypes. However, there is some suggestion that certain individuals with progressive non-syndromal dominant genetic hearing impairment may have disproportionately poor speech recognition for the degree of pure tone threshold elevation:

- acoustic reflex decay (ARD);
- other acoustic reflex measures;
- speech audiometry.

Chapter 7
Audiometric investigation of first-degree relatives

DAFYDD STEPHENS

Following a survey of current practice within the study group, the following set of tests was defined as the minimum set that should be performed on first-degree relatives of the proband under investigation.

First-degree relatives are the parents, children and siblings of the affected individuals, who share with them 50% of the same genes.

The following conclusions were reached with regard to *a minimum set of investigations.*

Tests should be applied to *both parents,* any *children* and all *siblings* of the *proband.* The aim is particularly to demonstrate any hearing loss that may be present. All branches of the family should be followed as far as possible. *Clinical examination* and tuning fork tests should be performed. *Békésy audiometry* 125 Hz–8 kHz should be conducted to define the audiometric configuration, with pure-tone audiometry at half-octave intervals conducted where that is not available.

The following tests would *not* normally be performed:

- pure tone audiometry – unless Békésy/Audioscan is not available; if tested, it should be performed at half-octave intervals;
- speech audiometry;
- auditory brainstem responses (ABR);
- acoustic reflex thresholds (ARTs);
- transient oto-acoustic emissions (TOAEs);
- extended high-frequency audiometry;
- vestibular tests – unless abnormalities are found in the proband.

Chapter 8
Audiometric investigation of carriers

DAFYDD STEPHENS, GENEVIÈVE LINA-GRANADE,
STAVROS HATZOPOULOS, FEI ZHAO

There has been an interest in the detection of subtle audiometric abnormalities in carriers of recessive and X-linked hearing impairment (e.g. parents, siblings and children of affected people) since the 1930s (Stephens and Francis, 1996).

A survey of study group members showed that few tests were being used systematically and that the test protocol for those tests that *were* being used differed from centre to centre.

Initially we considered tests that were being used but did not provide meaningful results, usually because of the range of abnormalities resulting from non-genetic factors. Subsequently certain tests were investigated by different members of the study group and rejected for similar reasons. The following recommendations were then made:

*The following tests should **not** normally be performed*

- pure-tone audiometry;
- acoustic reflex thresholds;
- extended high-frequency audiometry (>8,000 Hz);
- measures of frequency resolution;
- measures of temporal resolution;
- speech in noise tests.

The tests that merited further investigation were

- audioscan;
- distortion product oto-acoustic emissions (DPOAEs).

Due to the problems of relating the carrier results to a range of different genotypes, particulariy with non-syndromal recessive hearing impairment, these tests will be assessed further in carriers in whom the specific genotype has been confirmed. In both cases notches in the 500 Hz–3 kHz range have been taken as indicators of carrier status. A recent study (Zhao and Stephens, 1998) has shown a close relationship between notches obtained with the two techniques.

Audioscan – recommended protocol (see Zhao et al., 1998)

* Starting level – –5 dB HL
* Step size – 5 dB
* Sweep range – 300 Hz – 4,000 Hz
* Sweep rate – 30s/octave
* Pulsed tone – 2.5 pulses/s
* Ears tested – right then left

It is also important that the subject should receive some practice before starting on the test run.

DPOAEs – recommended protocol

This concerns the 2f1–f2 cubic distortion product otoacoustic emissions.

Protocol 1

* Stimulus levels – 70 dB and 70 dB SPL;
* frequency ratio (f1 : f2) – 1.22;
* step size – one-eighth of an octave;
* frequency range (geometric mean frequencies) – 1000 to 6000 Hz);
* number of stimulus averages – at least 48.

Protocol 2

* Stimulus levels – 60 dB and 50 dB SPL;
* frequency ratio (f1 : f2) – 1.22;
* step size – eight octave;
* frequency range (referred to F2) – 1000 to 6,000 Hz;
* number of stimulus averages – at least 48.

In addition, specific frequency testing with greater resolution around the frequency of the audioscan notches is being investigated.

Definitions of notches

Audioscan

- Depth 15 dB or more in either ear;
- frequency at maximum depth between 500 Hz and 3 kHz;
- width not considered;
- measures based on parameters defined by Laroche and Hétu (1997).

DPOAEs

- Depth 15 dB or more in either ear;
- deepest point – touching noise floor or 10 dB SPL.

References

Laroche C, Hétu R (1997) A study of the reliability of automatic audiometry by the frequency scanning method (Audioscan). Audiology 36: 1–18.

Stephens D, Francis M (1996) The detection of carriers of genetic hearing loss. In Martini A, Read A, Stephens D (eds) Genetics and Hearing Impairment. London: Whurr, pp. 100–8.

Zhao F, Stephens D (1998) Analyses of notches in Audioscan and DPOAEs in subjects with normal hearing. Audiology 37: 335–43.

Zhao F, Stephens D, Meredith R, Newton VE (1998) Audioscan notches in carriers of genetic hearing impairment. In Stephens D, Read A, Martini A (eds) Developments in Genetic Hearing Impairment. London: Whurr, pp. 60–7.

Chapter 9
Vestibular protocol

CLAES MÖLLER, LINDA LUXON, PATRICK HUYGEN, LARS ÖDKVIST, FLORIS WUYTS

The following protocol for the vestibular assessment of probands with genetic hearing impairment was developed by the vestibular working group of the Concerted Action project. It should be completed for each affected proband, and also family members when the proband is shown to be affected.

It comprises a minimal set of tests and does not preclude the addition of further investigations.

Anamnesis

Date of test
_____ dd/mm/yy
Date of birth
_____ dd/mm/yy
Sex
m/f
When was the child able to **walk** without help   _____ months

Problems with
  Walking in darkness   yes/ no/ unknown
  Walking on uneven surface or in sand   yes/ no/ unknown
  Gymnastics and sport activities   yes/ no/ unknown
  Motion sickness   yes/ no/ unknown
  Reading (visual fixation) during walking   yes/ no/ unknown
  Age of onset of vestibular problems   _____ years

36

Vestibular symptoms

Acute attacks of vertigo
    Character: rotational, linear, other_____
    Duration of symptoms (1: <1 month, 2: <6 months, 3: <1 year, 4:>1 year)
    Length of an attack (1: <5 min, 2: <20 min, 3: <2 hrs, 4: <12 hrs; 5: <24 hrs;
    6: >24 Hrs)
    Frequency of attack (1: once a year; 2: twice a year; 3: once a month; 4: once a
    week; 5: more frequent)
    Associated symptoms: tinnitus, fluctuating hearing loss, nausea, prolonged
    imbalance, other_____

Lateropulsion (tendency to fall sideways)	yes/ no/ unknown
Lightheadedness / faintness	yes/ no/ unknown
Unsteadiness / drunken feeling	yes/ no/ unknown
Oscillopsia (unsteady visual image/field)	
Unassociated with head movement	yes/ no/ unknown
Head movement induced	yes/ no/ unknown

History

Trauma including whiplash	yes/ no/ unknown
Infection (e.g. meningitis)	yes/ no/ unknown
Ototoxic drugs	yes/ no/ unknown
Perinatal problems (>48 hrs in SCBU-incubator)	yes/ no/ unknown

Family history: family members with balance dysfunction   yes/ no/ unknown
    Specify who, and what _____

Clinical examination

Ear, nose and throat examination   Normal/ Abnormal
Specify if abnormal
Cranial nerve examination   Normal/ Abnormal
Specify if abnormal
Wide based gait (eyes closed)   yes/ no

Nystagmus detection
    Spontaneous nystagmus (on direct observation)   yes/ no
        Patient seated looking in primary gaze position
    Spontaneous nystagmus (using Frenzles or goggles)   yes/ no
    Gaze-evoked nystagmus (30 degrees left–right from mid-position –   yes/ no
        naked eye)
    Positional nystagmus (lateral horizontal position)   yes/ no
    Head-shaking nystagmus (using Frenzles or goggles)   yes/ no
    Fistula test (pressure in the ear canal)   yes/ no/ unknown

Testing

Spontaneous nystagmus present in darkness: yes/ no
    left-right beating; slow phase velocity _____ (deg/s)
Positional nystagmus (lateral horizontal position) in darkness: yes/ no
    left-right beating; slow phase velocity _____ (deg/s)
Caloric testing (Bithermal-Binaural (250cc)) by preference and **for age>4 years**
    In darkness   yes/ no
    Right 30°C (Maximal slow phase velocity)   _____ deg/s
    Left 30°C   _____ deg/s
    Left 44°C   _____ deg/s
    Right 44°C   _____ deg/s

Bilateral hypoactivity   yes/ no
(if total sum of four irrigations <40 deg/sec in the dark, or if response
is below own normative limits)
If hypoactive: is the patient bilateral areflexive?   yes/ no
(choose one of the following)
Tap water calorics (___ °C) during 60 seconds irrigation – nystagmus present?
                                                                yes/ no
Ice water calorics (20 seconds) – nystagmus present?   yes/ no

Labyrinthine asymmetry:
$[(LW+LC) - (RW+RC)]/[LW+RW+LC+RC] \times 100 =$ _____ %

Nystagmus preponderance:
$[(LW+RC) - (LC+RW)]/[LW+RW+LC+RC] \times 100 =$ _____ %

Recording mode of eye movements
    Electro-oculography (electro-nystagmography)   yes/ no
    Video-oculography   yes/ no
    Other _____

For children <4 years or those not co-operative with the above assessment, the presence or absence of vestibular function should be assessed by a rotational test in the dark, evaluating the nystagmus response.

[Mark with a vertical line]
No response |_____| Normal nystagmus

Summary vestibular diagnosis

Vestibular activity: **Normal**
                                        Unilateral hypoactive left
                                        Unilateral hypoactive right
                                        Unilateral absent left

Unilateral absent right
Bilateral hypoactive
Bilateral absent
Central involvement

If more advanced equipment is available, a standard ENG/rotational protocol for the individual unit should be carried out and the results, together with normative data, valid for the laboratory, should be faxed with the basic vestibular assessment to Claes Möller, fax +46-31-82-9811, e-mail Claes.moller@audiology.gu.se, or Linda Luxon, fax +44-207-813-8107, e-mail linda.luxon@gosh-tr.nthames.nhs.uk

Chapter 10
Protocol for epidemiological studies on genetic hearing impairment

AGNETE PARVING, ADRIAN DAVIS

Background

In a previous EEC survey comprising the 1969 birth cohort, an estimated prevalence of 0.9/1,000 children with hearing impairment >50 dB HL for the better hearing ear, averaged across 0.5–4 kHz (BEHL 0.5–4 kHz) was found. Of these, 9% were ascribed to heredity (Martin et al., 1981). More recent studies from various countries and local areas in Europe have demonstrated a proportion of 30–50% of hereditary hearing impairment (Parving, 1995).

However, differences in hearing levels and lack of defined cohorts preclude valid comparisons or aggregation of data within the European countries. Prevalence estimates of hereditary hearing impairment in both children and adults are necessary in order to provide appropriate services for people with hearing impairment due to genetic factors, in terms of both diagnosis and counselling.

Some information on the proportion of children with hereditary hearing impairment in the European countries could be derived from the previous EEC survey (Martin et al., 1981) but the information was too limited and no information on the prevalence of genetic hearing impairment in adults was available. The interactions between endogenous and exogenous factors causing hearing impairment in adults are an important and a developing issue that should be highlighted in order to target people who are especially susceptible to environmental factors damaging the hearing organ (such as noise, ototoxic drugs and infections).

A standardized protocol is necessary in order to provide reliable information of this kind. This was defined by the study group on epidemiology of genetic hearing impairment and is described below.

Hearing level criteria in children – Permanent childhood hearing impairment may be defined as ≥ 50 dB in the better hearing ear, averaged across 0.5–4 kHz (BEHL 0.5–4 kHz).

Hereditary hearing impairment in children – Surveys of the proportions of different causative factors demonstrated substantial inconsistencies in the criteria for diagnosing a hereditary hearing impairment. Consequently criteria for hereditary hearing impairment were established and agreed. They are as shown in Table 10.1.

Table 10.1: Criteria for hereditary hearing impairment

1. One or both parents/grandparents affected.
2. Two or more generations affected.
3. Pedigree suggesting inheritance.
4. Two or more children with unaffected parents.
5. Consanguinity to any degree.
6. Only child with unaffected parents but with affected cousin(s).
   or
7. Pedigree indicating X-linked inheritance.
8. Pedigree indicating mitochondrial inheritance;
9. Recognized syndrome.

Based on the data from a questionnaire and the uniform criteria for inheritance, data from seven countries/local areas in Europe have been obtained showing a proportion of inheritance between 22% and 56% in the birth cohorts 1985–9 with BEHL 0.5–4 kHz ≥ 50 dB. Thus a highly preliminary prevalence estimate of 30–35/100,000 children suffering from hereditary hearing impairment could be obtained (Parving et al., 1998).

A proportion of unknown causes of hearing impairment, varying between 22% and 40% was demonstrated. This resulted in the development of a protocol for aetiological evaluation, in order to improve the quality of the diagnostic services within the EU. Minimum requirements for the protocol were agreed upon defining the aetiological evaluation as an ongoing long-term process as part of a surveillance programme. The minimum requirements are listed in Table 10.2.

The birth cohorts 1985–9 were subjected to this protocol, resulting in a proportion of inheritance of 28% to 56% with a proportion among these of non-syndromal hereditary hearing impairment of 66% to 94% and syndromal inheritance ranging from 6% to 34%.

Table 10.2: Minimal requirements for aetiological investigations

1. Thorough clinical evaluation but not necessarily referral to a paediatrician.
2. Thorough ENT examination including vestibular testing at an appropriate age.
3. Ophthalmological referral at the time of identification to an ophthalmologist, who is aware of the associations between hearing impairment and ophthalmological signs/symptoms.
4. CT/MRI scan at an appropriate age.
5. Urinalysis at the time of identification and repeated after at least the age of 10.
6. ECG at least once at an appropriate age.
7. Thyroid function tests (whatever available and decided by the individual physician) at an appropriate age.
8. Serological testing (dependent on history) before the age of 1 year.

The proportion of unknown cause ranges from 17% to 51%, and thus, the protocol does not seem to cause uniform improvements in the diagnostic evaluation. However, a one-and-a-half to two-year period is insufficient for diagnostic evaluation of hearing-impaired children. Moreover, previous studies have illustrated that a systematic evaluation protocol as part of a surveillance programme in hearing-impaired children can reduce the proportion of unknown causes (Parving, 1984; France and Stephens, 1995).

It should be emphasized that the clinical professional investigations included in the protocol are fundamental for aetiological diagnosis, which demands extensive collaboration from the parents. In order to improve the quality of the diagnostic evaluation, it is suggested that screening for known gene mutations causing hearing impairment should be included in the protocol. The 35 del G mutation of Connexin 26 is reported to be the most frequent in recessive non-syndromal hearing impairment, and screening for mutations in this gene might be included in the protocol, although screening for other genes such as Pendrin, COCH, Myosin 7A, and transcription factors known to cause hereditary hearing impairment may also be included. The promotion of molecular genetic methods is important in order to increase their availability as a laboratory service, offered to the clinicians as part of the hearing health services directed towards hearing-impaired people.

Hereditary hearing impairment in adults

Hearing impairment affects 18% to 20% of the adult population, and it is considered a major public heath problem. In view of the substantial lack of information about genetic factors causing hearing impairment in adults and their interaction with environmental factors causing hearing impairment, surveys of hereditary hearing impairment in adults were intended. Although prevalence estimates should be based on population studies, it was recognized that the time frame of the HEAR project could not meet this requirement.

References

France EA, Stephens SDG (1995) All Wales audiology and genetic service for hearing-impaired young adults. Journal of Audiological Medicine 4: 67–84.

Martin JAM, Bentzen O, Colley JRT, Hennebert D, Holm C, Iurato S, deJonge A, McCullen O, Meyer ML, Moore WJ, Morgan A (1981) Childhood deafness in the European Community. Scandinavian Audiology 10: 165–74.

Parving A (1984) Aetiological diagnosis in hearing impaired children. Clinical value and application of a modern examination progamme. International Journal of Pediatric Otorhinolaryngology 7: 29–38.

Parving A (1995) Factors causing hearing impairment – some perspectives from Europe. Journal of the American Academy of Audiology 6: 387–95.

Parving A (Co-ordinator), Admiraal R, Apaydin F, Arslan E, Davis A, Dias O, Fortnum H, Grisanti G, Gross M, Hess M, Konrádsson K, Lina-Granade G, Mäki-Torkko E, Newton V, O'Donovan C, Orzan E, Sorri M, Stephens SDG, Tsakinokos MD, Waagenaar M, Wezl-Müller K (1998) Epidemiology of hereditary hearing impairment in childhood – preliminary estimates from the European Union. In Martini A, Read A, Stephens D (eds) Developments in Genetic Hearing Impairment. London: Whurr, pp. 35–42.

Chapter 11
The European Congenital Ear Anomaly Inventory

PAUL VAN DE HEYNING, FRANK DECLAU,
ALESSANDRO MARTINI, COR CREMERS

Introduction

Many classifications have been proposed in order to define congenital ear pathology. The rationale for classification is manifold. It can aim at a meaningful organization of knowledge such as presentation in an ascending order of severity, or a lumping into categories of common embryological or developmental aetiology or heredity. It can enhance communication between clinicians.

The European Congenital Ear Anomaly Inventory (ECEAI) represents the classification system of congenital ear anomalies, as proposed by the European HEAR project (Hereditary Deafness, Epidemiology and Clinical Research, BIOMED 2 Concerted Action). It aims at a comprehensive and systematic anatomical description of the different components of the ear. This classification system is not linked to a particular aetiology. It emphasizes the necessity of evaluating all the different parts of the auditory system from the auricle to the external auditory canal, the middle ear, the inner ear, the internal auditory canal and the central auditory nervous system (CANS). The evaluation should be based on clinical investigations as well as on imaging techniques.

This inventory contains and unites a number of existing classification systems of the constituent parts.

Aim of the classification

The proposed classification aims to enhance communication between clinicians by describing anomalies as precisely as possible, irrespective of the aetiology or influence. It therefore uses an anatomical descriptive approach of the different constituent parts of the ear and the auditory system – the auricle, the external auditory canal, the middle ear, the inner ear including the cochlea and labyrinthine system, the internal auditory canal and the central auditory nervous system.

It has been observed, in many reports and studies, that all types of combinations of anomalies of the different parts can occur in an individual patient. The finding of an anomaly in one part even enhances the likelihood of the existence of another anomaly in one of the other parts of the ear.

This basic observation warrants the development of an inventory. Hence the classification system was called the European Congenital Ear Anomaly Inventory (ECEAI).

The basis for the reporting of the anomalies is clinical observation together with CT and MRI imaging.

The general terminology and definitions as proposed by the HEAR project were implemented for the congenital ear anomalies.

The European Congenital Ear Anomaly Inventory (ECEAI)

For each element of the ECEAI, the group evaluated whether a recommendation or a guideline for classification could be made. Indeed many classifications have been developed from a particular aetiological viewpoint, as tools for a specific research purpose, or are linked to a particular surgical technique. Other classification systems lack a scientific basis. Some elements lack of knowledge prevents meaningful organization.

Classification of auricular malformations

The classification recommended was proposed by Weerda and Siegert (1998). The system classifies the anomalies by increasing degree of severity and increasing number of surgical procedures to correct the anomalies. Three degrees are used according to Marx (1926):

First-degree dysplasia.

- General definition: most structures of a normal auricle are recognizable.
- Surgical definition: reconstruction does not require use of additional tissues.

Second-degree dysplasia.

• General definition: some structures of a normal auricle are recognizable.
• Surgical definition: partial reconstruction requires additional skin and cartilage.

Third-degree dysplasias and anotia.

• General definition: none of the structures of a normal auricle are recognizable.
• Surgical definition: total reconstruction requires the use of skin and large amounts of cartilage.

External ear canal

A congenital ear anomaly is called 'major' when the external ear canal is atretic. The desciptions 'major' and 'minor' were linked to the reconstructive possibilities in earlier days. Such classification into major and minor has lost its relevance due to new techniques such as the bone anchored epithesis and bone anchored hearing aid (Granström et al., 1993, 1997). Nevertheless, classification in terms of major and minor (middle) ear anomalies is retained mainly for historical reasons and because this description is generally accepted.

For an overview of the role played by the external ear canal in the former classifications, see Declau et al. (1999).

Minor anomalies of the ossicular chain

The classification of ossicular anomalies has undergone many changes over time. Based on an extensive literature review (Charachon, 1994; Morisseau-Durand et al., 1994; Hara et al., 1997; Causse, 1997) and on analysis of many cases by Tos, the following classification was developed, which originates from the Cremers' classification (Teunissen and Cremers, 1993). This classification acts as the HEAR guideline for minor ossicular anomalies. For the detailed work with a schematic representation, we refer to Tos (1999).

Type I : Congenital stapes ankylosis*
        a: footplate fixed with monopodal or normal suprastructure
        b: suprastructure fixed

Type II : the same plus another ossicular chain anomaly*
        a: discontinuity
        b: epitympanic fixation
        c: tympanic fixation (malleus handle or/and long process)

Type III: Congenital anomaly of the ossicular chain but a mobile stapes footplate
    a: discontinuity
    b: epitympanic fixation
    c: tympanic fixation (malleus handle or/and long process)

Type IV: Congenital aplasia or severe dysplasia of the oval or round window *
    aplasia
    dysplasia
    – crossing VII nerve
    – persistent stapedial artery

*stapedial tendon absent

Inner ear anomalies

At present the classification following Jackler et al. (1987) is recommended:

A. An absent or malformed cochlea
1. Complete labyrinthine aplasia (Michel deformity).
2. Cochlear aplasia: no cochlea, normal or malformed vestibule and semicircular canals.
3. Cochlear hypoplasia: small cochlear bud, normal or malformed vestibule and semicircular canals.
4. Incomplete partition (classical Mondini): small cochlea with incomplete or no interscalar septum, normal or malformed vestibule and semicircular canals.
5. Common cavity: cochlea and vestibule form a common cavity without internal architecture; normal or malformed semicircular canals.

B With a normal cochlea
1. Vestibule-lateral semicircular canal dysplasia: enlarged vestibule with a short, dilated lateral semicircular canal; the remaining semicircular canals are normal.
2. Enlarged vestibular aqueduct accompanied by normal semicircular canals, normal or enlarged vestibule

It should be noted, however, that recent advances in imaging have revealed that combinations of inner ear anomalies exist that cannot be classified following the above system (Triglia, 1993). This has become particularly obvious on studying enlarged vestibular aqueduct syndromes (Lemmerling et al., 1997). New ideas are arising and will eventually lead to a renewal of the classification of inner ear and CANS deformities (Smith and Harker, 1998).

Internal auditory canal and the central auditory nervous system

The currently available classification of observed anomalies in the internal auditory canal is from Casselman et al. (1997). Many case reports are emerging on observed congenital anomalies of the CANS. Application of fMRI techniques and PETscan will alter our understanding of the CANS. Increased knowledge of genetic control of the development of the CANS will also dramatically influence our approach to anomalies. Therefore no generally accepted classification system is currently available. It is, however, recommended that the description of the internal auditory canal and its content as well as the CANS be included in the inventory. Immediate consequences may arise from this evaluation in the field of cochlear implantation.

Complications of congenital anomalies of the ear

The study group highlights the risk of the following complications in cases of congenital ear anomalies.

Cerebro-spinal fluid leak and otogenic meningitis
    Surgical: presents as gusher
    Spontaneous
        LSCC and vestibule enlarged or confluent
        No internal structure in the cochlea (Scheibe)
        Route through IAC and basal turn (X linked)
        Enlarged cochlear aqueduct
        Fistula in stapes footplate
        Congenital cholesteatoma
        Surgical risk of facial palsy

Conclusion

The classification of congenital ear anomalies is based on an anatomical decriptive inventory of the different parts of the ear, and not on a list of combinations of anomalies of the different elements: auricle, external auditory canal, middle ear, inner ear, internal auditory canal and the CANS.

It is recognized that different combinations of structures can be involved, and that this is even frequent. Hence these combinations have to be actively sought.

Acknowledgements

Group IVb of HEAR was dedicated to otological malformations and connected surgical problems. The study group consisted of M Amadori,

J Casselman, JB Causse, R Charachon, C Cremers, F Declau, G Granström, A Martini, M Tos, T Somers, FE Offeciers, P van de Heyning and was advised by H Weerda. The authors are grateful to their colleagues for their valuable contribution to the work described here.

References

Casselman JW, Offeciers FE, Govaerts P, Kuhweide EW, Geldof H, Somers T, D'Hont G (1997) Aplasia and hypoplasia of the vestibulocochlear nerve: diagnosis with MR imaging. Radiology 202: 773–81.

Causse JB (1997) Gratacap Minor ossicular anomalies. In: The OTO-ROM Colombiers Services. Colombiers.

Charachon R, Barthez M, Lavieille J-P (1994) Les malformations mineures de la chaine ossiculaire. Annales d'Oto-laryngologie et Chirurgie Cervicofaciale. (Paris) 111: 69–74.

Declau F, Cremers C, Van de Heyning P (1999) Diagnosis and management strategies in congenital atresia of the external auditory canal. British Journal of Audiology 33: 313–27.

Granström G, Bergstrom K, Tjellstrom A (1993) The bone-anchored hearing aid and bone-anchored epithesis for congenital ear malformations. Otolaryngology and Head and Neck Surgery 109: 46–53.

Hara A, Ase Y, Kusakri J, Kurosaki Y (1997) Dominant hereditary conductive hearing loss due to an ossified stapedius tendon. Archives of Otolaryngology and Head and Neck Surgery 123: 1133–5.

Jackler R, Luxford W, House WF (1987) Congenital malformations of the inner ear: a classification based on embryogenesis. Laryngoscope 97 Suppl 40: 2–14.

Lemmerling MM, Mancuso AA, Antonelli PJ, Kubilis PS (1997) Normal modiolus: CT appearance in patients with a large vestibular aqueduct. Radiology 204: 213–19.

Morisseau-Durand MP, Ayache D, Simon D, Manach Y, Roulleau P (1994) Aplasie mineure de l'oreille. Annales d'Oto-laryngologie et Chirurgie Cervicofaciale (Paris) 111: 470–5.

Smith SD, Harker L (1998) Single gene influences on radiologically-detectable malformations of the inner ear. Journal of Communication Disorders 31: 391–410.

Teunissen E, Cremers C (1993) Annals of Otology; Rhinology and Laryngology 102: 606–12.

Tos M (1999) Congenital ossicular fixations and defects. In Tos M (1999) Manual of Middle Ear Surgery. Vol. 4, Chapter 11. Stuttgart: Georg Thieme Verlag.

Triglia JM, Nicollas R, Ternier F, Cannoni M (1993) Deafness caused by malformation of the inner ear. Current contribution of x-ray computed tomography. Annales d'Oto-laryngologie et Chirurgie Cervicofaciale (Paris) 110: 241–6.

Weerda H, Siegert R (1998) Classification of auricular malformations. Face 5: 157–8.

Chapter 12
Protocol for syndromal disorders associated with hearing impairment

ELISA CALZOLARI, ALBERTO SENSI, FRANCESCA GUALANDI

Introduction

In recent years hearing impairment associated with cranio-facial malformations has been the focus of several research studies that led to the identification of some genes responsible for common disorders (Waardenburg and Treacher Collins Syndromes).

Cranio-facial malformations represent a difficult task for the clinician (surgical programming, rehabilitation and so forth). Furthermore, in most cases it is difficult to differentiate between cranio-facial syndromes due to genetic and other causes and this is extremely important for 'counselling'. All types of syndromal deafness, although representing a large percentage of genetic hearing impairment, present low relative frequencies, so that international co-operation is necessary for an adequate study.

Syndromal diagnosis is a difficult task for many reasons:

- the *rarity* of most of these conditions precludes a direct experience of the majority of them;
- *heterogeneity* – a single phenotype may be a consequence of different pathogenetic and etiologic events;
- *pleiotropy* – term meaning that a single gene may cause many different phenotypic effects, often apparently unrelated pathogenetically;
- *non-specificity* of individual defects;
- wide *variability* of clinical expression;
- absence in most cases of a unique *specific and sensitive test*.

Of course, the rarity of many types of syndromal HL means that they can be dealt with adequately only with recourse to authoritative texts (Jones,

1988; Buyse, 1990; Gorlin et al., 1995; Gorlin et al., 1990; Stevenson et al., 1993) and databases (POSSUM; Oxford Medical Database), whereas pleiotropy implies that a multidisciplinary approach is often required to achieve a complete view of these complex clinical pictures.

With rare exceptions, a clinical diagnosis of a pattern of malformations cannot be made on the basis of a single defect. It usually depends on the detection of the overall pattern of anomalies. Recognition of minor defects may be as helpful as recognition of major anomalies in this regard.

The variability of clinical expression is so wide in most syndromal HL that hearing impairment may constitute the main or apparently the only problem in some subjects, and the prominent involvement of other organs or systems may sometimes obscure HL in others. Waardenburg syndrome type II is a good example of expression variability: affected subjects may present bilaterally profound HL with only minimal hypopigmentation findings, whereas relatives may show classic heterochromia iridis/iridium, white forelock, but normal audiometry or only minimal or unilateral hypoacusis. In these cases only the examination of the whole family can allow the correct diagnosis to be made (Sensi et al., 1994). Moreover, the complete expression of the syndromal phenotype may be age dependent so that HL may be detected well before other symptoms, such as retinitis pigmentosa in Usher syndrome or goitre in Pendred syndrome. In these cases, a careful systematic search for the early subclinical manifestations, repeated over the years, can lead to the correct diagnosis.

On the other hand, HL may develop very late and sometimes it is detected just because a particular syndrome is suspected. Indeed, it is common in Alport syndrome to find subjects in whom HL is clinically evident after renal involvement has already caused renal failure. Similarly, in Vohwinkel syndrome (mutilating keratoderma), the palmoplantar keratosis is evident from the first months of life, but HL may be mild even in adulthood (Sensi et al., 1994). In these cases the involvement of other organs is evident but the relation between the first disease and HL may be missed.

Thus the problem of syndromal HL diagnosis has two aspects:

- not to miss the syndromal nature of HL when only subclinical involvement of other systems or subtle dysmorphological elements are recognizable, and
- to diagnose complex clinical pictures correctly.

For the first aim a systematic approach is required with a standard screening procedure targeted at the syndromal HL conditions. Obviously, the approach must be adapted to the age and the general condition of patients.

Leaving out the specific audiological and vestibular examinations, we mention here the anamnestic, physical, laboratory and specialist evaluations that we generally include in the screening procedure (Table 12.1).

Clinical history and pedigree analysis

A detailed family history, including at least three generations of family members, has to be collected. The pedigree analysis differs from a simple family history not only because of the methodology used to collect the data but especially because it implies a familial approach to the diagnosis.

It is worth noting that syndromal HL may or may not be genetic (monogenic, polygenic mitochondrial or chromosomal) and that negative pedigrees are commonly found in both cases. Consanguinity and even remote family history of early onset or late onset of HL have to be sought and significant medical or physical features in deaf individuals or relatives (such as pigmentary alteration), structural anomalies (ear, cardiovascular, skeletal) evaluated. Photographs of other affected relatives for whom personal examination is not possible may prove helpful.

A pregnancy history has to be taken, concentrating particularly on prenatal exposure, prenatal events and postnatal events, and serological test performed during pregnancy should be recorded.

Specific diagnostic examinations

An ECG for QT evaluation should be always obtained in order to rule out the Jervell Nielsen syndrome, an autosomal recessive condition, characterized by possible fainting attacks during which the affected subjects may die.

Although the specific test for Pendred syndrome diagnosis is the perchlorate test, the TSH and fT4 determination together with physical

Table 12.1: Screening standard procedure

- Specific clinical history (with pregnancy serologic documentation);
- dysmorphologic evaluation;
- pedigree analysis (with audiometric examination of all the first-degree relatives);
- ophthalmologic examination;
- ECG;
- TSH and fT4;
- creatinine and urea nitrogen;
- venous blood pH;
- electrolytes;
- urine standard analysis.

examination of the neck can be considered a satisfactory screening procedure for practical clinical purposes.

Specialist ophthalmologic evaluation should be always performed with indirect fundoscopy for retinal periphery and slit lamp examination. The examination is relevant not only for the detection of retinitis pigmentosa or optic atrophy, but also for congenital infections that very often reveal themselves as peripheral chorioretinal reliquates or lens opacifications. Cataracts are also seen in many metabolic conditions.

A psychomotor and neurologic evaluation can be approached at a non-specialist level in a screening schedule, although the difficulties in assessing mental retardation by a non-specialist may be relevant in deaf children. Moreover, possible delays in walking may raise suspicions of vestibular involvement.

Urine sediment, creatinine, blood pH and serum electrolyte anomalies can allow the detection of subjects who need to undergo further evaluations for eventual diagnosis of conditions associating renal disease to HL.

A cytogenetic examination may be required after dysmorphologic evaluation.

Special procedures or targeted re-examination may be requested after one or more specific diagnostic hypotheses have been made. Reference to authoritative databases or texts is mandatory in this case.

Dysmorphologic examination

A detailed description of physical examination with particular regard to the most relevant elements in syndromal HL is essential for the formulation of a specific diagnosis and genetic counselling.

A dysmorphological evaluation requires a good knowledge of 'normality' and its variations and specific information about embryological development and its aberrations. Many minor abnormalities or variants may result, which are of relevance only in the whole context of a diagnostic hypothesis and taking into account familial and racial characteristics. Detailed descriptions and tables of normal physical measurements will be found in Aase (1990), Gorlin et al. (1990), Gorlin et al. (1995), Hall et al. (1989), Jones (1988), Stevenson et al. (1993).

A systematic, precise and homogeneous collection of dysmorphologic data is needed for diagnostic purposes, for the study of phenotypic variability and for the delineation of new syndromes. In this regard a specific detailed clinical form has been prepared by the fourth study group on craniofacial malformations and hearing impairment for clinical geneticists. A questionnaire has also been studied for ENT and other specialists for a preliminary screening of deaf probands.

Objective of the study

The objective of the study was to improve knowledge of the anomalies/syndromes that include hearing impairment and malformations of first and second branchial arches, to facilitate the provision of a better service to parents and families.

Specific objectives of the study are:

- to study the phenotypic variability with particular interest to inter- and intra-familial variability;
- delineation of new syndromes;
- identification of possible environmental factors influencing or causing the anomalies;
- evaluation of familial cases.

Results of the application of the protocol and clinical form in Ferrara

The screening protocol and clinical form were applied to 236 deaf probands and families, referred to the Audiological Department or to the Genetic Service. Fifty-eight families were enrolled during the period 1997–8; all the other cases were evaluated retrospectively.

The classification of deaf probands obtained by the systematic utilization of the protocol is summarized in Table 12.2. The genetic conditions diagnosed represent 49.5% of the whole series. The high proportion of genetic conditions found can probably be explained by two factors:

- the deafness referred to the genetic service is clearly selected as recurrent;
- the systematic examination allowed the recognition of genetic forms previously undetected.

In our survey, the proportion of syndromic conditions (including Mendelian, non-Mendelian, chromosomal and environmental conditions in the TORCH complex) reaches 27%. It is worth noticing that 18% of cases were labelled as 'non-classified associated findings'; this group probably includes rare syndromic conditions that the protocol did not specifically define. In most cases other specific investigations were prescribed. The theoretical proportion of syndromes in congenital HL is about 30%, but in postlingual HL it is considerably lower. Our survey includes postlingual HL, so the proportion of 27% of syndromal conditions is higher than expected and is probably due to sample selection and perhaps to the systematic dysmorphologic approach.

PROTOCOL

Centre reporting the case .... Centre code ....

Proband code .... diagnosis...

Slides or prints taken   NO ❑   YES ❑   proband DNA sample taken   NO ❑   YES ❑

Cell line   NO ❑   YES ❑   family DNA samples taken   NO ❑   YES ❑

birthplace ....   birth date ....sex   F ❑   M ❑

Paternal history
birthplace ....   birth date....................................

noise exposure   NO ❑   YES ❑   ....
mutagens exposure   NO ❑   YES ❑   ....
deafness/hypoacusis   NO ❑   YES ❑   ....
audiometry performed   NO ❑   YES ❑
audiological findings...
....
other known diseases ....
dysmorphologic examination: performed   NO ❑   YES ❑

Maternal history
birthplace ....   birth date....................................

noise exposure   NO ❑   YES ❑   ....
mutagens exposure   NO ❑   YES ❑   ....
deafness/hypoacusis   NO ❑   YES ❑   ....
audiometry performed   NO ❑   YES ❑
audiological findings...
....
other known diseases ....
dysmorphologic examination: performed   NO ❑   YES ❑

Proband gestation
duration weeks ....   weight gain ....   fetal activity ....

infections in pregnancy   NO ❑   YES ❑   ....
TORCH serology available   NO ❑   YES ❑
alcohol   NO ❑   YES ❑   mean daily intake ....
drugs in pregnancy   NO ❑   YES ❑   specify the drug/s, the intake, the period of exposure:
....
....
....

other problems in   NO ❑   YES ❑
pregnancy
....
....
....

Proband birth

mode ......   birth weight ....   birth length ....   birth OFC ....

jaundice   NO ❑   YES ❑ specify history..
....

anoxia   NO ❑   YES ❑ specify history..
....

trauma   NO ❑   YES ❑ specify history: ....
....
....

apgar score ....

other problems at birth   NO ❑   YES ❑ specify: ....
....
....

Proband history

General health..
....

Previous serious illness   NO ❑   YES ❑ specify: ....

Meningoencephalitis   NO ❑   YES ❑ specify: ....
....

Hospitalization   NO ❑   YES ❑ specify history: ....
....
....

Exposition to ototoxic agents

         drugs   NO ❑   YES ❑ specify: ....
....

         infection   NO ❑   YES ❑ specify: ....
....

         noise   NO ❑   YES ❑ specify: ....
....

Growth..
....

Developmental progress

normal psychomotor development   YES ❑   NO ❑ specify.....................................
....

holding head   NO ❑   YES ❑ *age*..
sitting   NO ❑   YES ❑ *age*..
standing   NO ❑   YES ❑ *age*...
walking   NO ❑   YES ❑ *age*..
speech present   NO ❑   YES ❑
lallation   NO ❑   YES ❑ *age*..
single words   NO ❑   YES ❑ *age*..
words in sentences   NO ❑   YES ❑ *age*..
behaviour...
....
....

age of onset of deafness..
rate of progression of deafness..

suspected causative event...
....

Pedigree
(it is recommended that first degree relatives are evaluated with at least recommended puretone audiometry and general physical evaluation)

legend

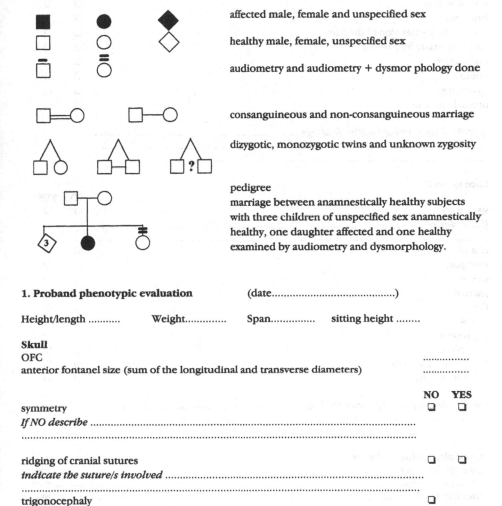

affected male, female and unspecified sex

healthy male, female, unspecified sex

audiometry and audiometry + dysmor phology done

consanguineous and non-consanguineous marriage

dizygotic, monozygotic twins and unknown zygosity

pedigree
marriage between anamnestically healthy subjects with three children of unspecified sex anamnestically healthy, one daughter affected and one healthy examined by audiometry and dysmorphology.

1. Proband phenotypic evaluation   (date..)

Height/length .... Weight.............. Span............... sitting height ....

Skull
OFC   ....
anterior fontanel size (sum of the longitudinal and transverse diameters)   ....

	NO	YES
symmetry	❏	❏

If NO describe ....
....

| ridging of cranial sutures | ❏ | ❏ |

indicate the suture/s involved ....
....

trigonocephaly	❏	
fs24 ❏		
brachycephaly	❏	❏
scaphocephaly	❏	❏
turricephaly	❏	❏
high forehead	❏	❏
prominent forehead	❏	❏
sloping forehead	❏	❏
normal cranial shape	❏	❏
other..	❏	❏

....

Scalp   NO   YES
generalized alopecia   ❏   ❏
low posterior hairline   ❏   ❏
upswept posterior hairline   ❏   ❏
low anterior hairline   ❏   ❏
widow's peak   ❏   ❏
baldness   ❏   ❏
lateral cheek extension of the hair   ❏   ❏
supernumerary hair whorl   ❏   ❏
scalp defects   ❏   ❏
poliosis   ❏   ❏
sparse hair   ❏   ❏
normal hair line   ❏   ❏

specific description of positive findings...
....
....

Face general

                                                   NO   YES
symmetry   ❏   ❏
if NO, describe...
....

round   ❏   ❏
elongated   ❏   ❏
broad   ❏   ❏
narrow   ❏   ❏
flat   ❏   ❏
coarse   ❏   ❏
expressionless   ❏   ❏
drooping   ❏   ❏
facial nerve paralysis   ❏   ❏
normal appearance   ❏   ❏

specific description of positive findings...
....
....

Periocular region and eyes
inner canthal distance   .... mm
interpupillary distance   .... mm
outer canthal distance   .... mm
                                                   NO   YES
Hypoplastic supraorbital ridges   ❏   ❏
Hyperplastic supraorbital ridges   ❏   ❏
orbital symmetry   ❏   ❏
strabismus   ❏   ❏
Duane phenomenon   ❏   ❏
downslanting palpebral fissures   ❏   ❏
upslanting palpebral fissures   ❏   ❏

		RIGHT		LEFT	
		NO	YES	NO	YES
normally oriented palpebral fissures			☐		☐
synophyris			☐		☐
eyebrows					
	sparse	☐	☐	☐	☐
	normal	☐	☐	☐	☐
	other	☐	☐	☐	☐
palpebral fissures shape	almond	☐	☐	☐	☐
	blepharophimosis	☐	☐	☐	☐
	entropion	☐	☐	☐	☐
	ectropion	☐	☐	☐	☐
	normal	☐	☐	☐	☐
lacrimal duct	stenosis	☐	☐	☐	☐
	atresia	☐	☐	☐	☐
	normal	☐	☐	☐	☐
upper lid	cleft	☐	☐	☐	☐
	epicanthic fold	☐	☐	☐	☐
	ptosis	☐	☐	☐	☐
	normal	☐	☐	☐	☐
eyelashes	deficit total or localized	☐	☐	☐	☐
	normal distribution	☐	☐	☐	☐
lower lid	cleft	☐	☐	☐	☐
	epicanthus inversus	☐	☐	☐	☐
	ectropion	☐	☐	☐	☐
	normal	☐	☐	☐	☐
eyelashes	deficit total or localized	☐	☐	☐	☐
	normal distribution	☐	☐	☐	☐
ocular globe	microphthalmos	☐	☐	☐	☐
	anophthalmos	☐	☐	☐	☐
	periocular tags	☐	☐	☐	☐
protrusion	protruding	☐	☐	☐	☐
	deep set	☐	☐	☐	☐
	normal	☐	☐	☐	☐
corneal diameter		....		....	
sclerae	colour	....		....	
	dermoids	☐	☐	☐	☐
irides	colour	....		....	
	coloboma	☐	☐	☐	☐
other		☐	☐	☐	☐

specific description of positive findings...
....
....

Midface and Nose

	NO	YES
midface hypoplasia	❏	❏
malar hypoplasia	❏	❏
flat premaxillary region	❏	❏
prominent premaxillary region	❏	❏

nose

		NO	YES
length	short	❏	❏
	long	❏	❏
	normal	❏	❏
shape	bulbous	❏	❏
	beaked	❏	❏
	tubular	❏	❏
	proboscis	❏	❏
	normal	❏	❏
root	low	❏	❏
	high	❏	❏
	broad	❏	❏
	normal	❏	❏
bridge	low	❏	❏
	broad	❏	❏
	high	❏	❏
	nasal pit	❏	❏
	normal	❏	❏
tip	bifid	❏	❏
	hypoplastic	❏	❏
	downturned	❏	❏
	upturned	❏	❏
	normal	❏	❏
nares	anteversed	❏	❏
	hypoplasic alae	❏	❏
	single nostril	❏	❏
	normal	❏	❏
columella	short	❏	❏
	thick	❏	❏
	normal	❏	❏
choanal	stenosis	❏	❏
	atresia	❏	❏
other		❏	❏

specific description of positive findings..
....
....

Perioral region

		NO	YES
mouth	macrostomia	☐	☐
	microstomia	☐	☐
	asymmetry	☐	☐
	downturned corners	☐	☐
	oblique facial clefts	☐	☐
	width	☐	☐
	normal	☐	☐
philtrum	length	....	
	smooth	☐	☐
	deep	☐	☐
	normal shape	☐	☐
upper lip	thin	☐	☐
	thick	☐	☐
	cleft right	☐	☐
	cleft left	☐	☐
	cleft central	☐	☐
	normal	☐	☐
lower lip	thin	☐	☐
	thick	☐	☐
	everted	☐	☐
	pit	☐	☐
	normal	☐	☐
mandible/chin	asymmetry	☐	☐
	micrognathia	☐	☐
	retrognathia	☐	☐
	macrognathia	☐	☐
	prognathia	☐	☐
	cleft	☐	☐
	chin creases	☐	☐
	temporo-mandibular joints abnormalities	☐	☐
	normal	☐	☐

specific description of positive findings...
....
....

Oral cavity

teeth

eruption   normal ❏   late   ❏   early ❏   not determined ❏

shape/size   normal ❏   abnormal ❏

	NO	YES
anodontia	❏	❏
oligodontia	❏	❏
crowding	❏	❏
malalignment	❏	❏
enamel defects	❏	❏
dentinogenesis imperfecta	❏	❏
diastema	❏	❏
single incisor	❏	❏

vestibulus

	NO	YES
aberrant frenula	❏	❏
normal frenula	❏	❏
absent Stensen's duct	❏	❏

tongue

	NO	YES
macroglossia	❏	❏
microglossia	❏	❏
glossoptosis	❏	❏
asymmetry	❏	❏
lobulated	❏	❏
normal	❏	❏

palate

	NO	YES
ogival	❏	❏
narrow	❏	❏
secondary alveolar ridges	❏	❏
agenesis of soft palate	❏	❏
immobile soft palate	❏	❏
normal	❏	❏

cleft

	NO	YES		
uvula bifida	❏	❏		
submucous	❏	❏		
anterior unilateral incomplete	❏	❏	right ❏	left ❏
anterior unilateral complete	❏	❏	right ❏	left ❏
anterior bilateral incomplete	❏	❏		
anterior bilateral complete	❏	❏		
posterior incomplete	❏	❏		
posterior complete	❏	❏		
posterior U shaped	❏	❏		

specific description of positive findings...
....
....

Ears

		RIGHT		LEFT	
		NO	YES	NO	YES
placement	low	❑	❑	❑	❑
	abnormal	❑	❑	❑	❑
	normal	❑	❑	❑	❑
rotation	posterior	❑	❑	❑	❑
	anterior	❑	❑	❑	❑
	normal (about 15°)	❑	❑	❑	❑
angulation from the head					
	increased (protruding)	❑	❑	❑	❑
	normal	❑	❑	❑	❑
size		.... mm		.... mm	
pinna shape	minor abnormalities	❑	❑	❑	❑
	microtia I	❑	❑	❑	❑
	lop	❑	❑	❑	❑
	lop-satyr	❑	❑	❑	❑
	cup	❑	❑	❑	❑
	microtia II	❑	❑	❑	❑
	microtia III	❑	❑	❑	❑
	anotia	❑	❑	❑	❑
	normal	❑	❑	❑	❑
lobe	large	❑	❑	❑	❑
	hypoplastic	❑	❑	❑	❑
	creased	❑	❑	❑	❑
	cleft	❑	❑	❑	❑
	normal	❑	❑	❑	❑
pits		❑	❑	❑	❑
tags		❑	❑	❑	❑
meatus	stenotic	❑	❑	❑	❑
	atretic	❑	❑	❑	❑
	normal	❑	❑	❑	❑

specific description of positive findings...
....
....

Neck

	NO	YES
short	❑	❑
asymmetric	❑	❑
branchial remnants	❑	❑
pterygium	❑	❑
enlarged thyroid	❑	❑
lateral cervical thymus	❑	❑
normal	❑	❑

specific description of positive findings...
....
....

Chest and shoulders

	NO	YES
pectus excavatum	❑	❑
pectus carinatum	❑	❑
shield chest	❑	❑
sloping shoulders	❑	❑
clavicle absence	❑	❑
pectoralis major absence	❑	❑
supernumerary nipples	❑	❑
absent/hypoplastic nipples	❑	❑
dextrocardia	❑	❑
heart murmurs	❑	❑
other abnormalities	❑	❑
normal	❑	❑
inter-nipple distance	.... cm	
chest circumference	.... cm	

specific description of positive findings...
....
....

Abdomen

	NO	YES
hepatomegaly	❑	❑
splenomegaly	❑	❑
inguinal hernia	❑	❑
umbilical hernia	❑	❑
umbilicus displacement	❑	❑
omphalocele	❑	❑
prune belly sequence	❑	❑
normal	❑	❑

specific description of positive findings...
....
....

Back	NO	YES
scoliosis	❑	❑
kyphosis	❑	❑
Sprengel abnormalities	❑	❑
winged scapulas	❑	❑
small scapulas	❑	❑
spina bifida	❑	❑
pilonidal sinus	❑	❑
normal	❑	❑

specific description of positive findings...
....
....

Genitals	NO	YES	
ambiguous genitalia	❑	❑	
hypospadias (if yes indicate grade)	❑	❑	....
epispadias	❑	❑	
extrophy of the bladder	❑	❑	
shawl scrotum	❑	❑	
bifid scrotum	❑	❑	
macrorchidism	❑	❑	
cryptorchidism	❑	❑	
testicular hypoplasia	❑	❑	
hypoplastic labia	❑	❑	
imperforate hymen	❑	❑	
vagina absent	❑	❑	
other	❑	❑	
normal	❑	❑	

specific description of positive findings...
....
....

Anus and perineum	NO	YES
displaced anus	❑	❑
anal atresia	❑	❑
imperforate anus	❑	❑
other	❑	❑
normal	❑	❑

specific description of positive findings...
....
....

Upper limbs	NO	YES
asymmetry	❑	❑
cubitus valgus	❑	❑
cubitus varus	❑	❑
elbow webbing	❑	❑
other joint abnormalities	❑	❑

		RIGHT		LEFT	
		NO	YES	NO	YES
shortening	rhizomelic	❑	❑	❑	❑
	mesomelic	❑	❑	❑	❑
	acromelic	❑	❑	❑	❑
homerus abnormalities		❑	❑	❑	❑
forearm abnormalities		❑	❑	❑	❑

specific description of positive findings..
....
....

Hands

		RIGHT		LEFT	
		NO	YES	NO	YES
general	total length	....		....	
	palm length	....		....	
	single crease	❑	❑	❑	❑
	abnormal palmar crease pattern	❑	❑	❑	❑
	palmar keratosis	❑	❑	❑	❑
	hyperextensibility	❑	❑	❑	❑
	absent hand	❑	❑	❑	❑
	split hand	❑	❑	❑	❑
	hypotrophic thenar eminence	❑	❑	❑	❑
	hypotrophic hypothenar eminence	❑	❑	❑	❑
	prominent finger pads	❑	❑	❑	❑
	nail abnormalities	❑	❑	❑	❑
thumb	broad	❑	❑	❑	❑
	absent-hypoplastic	?	?	?	?
	triphalangeal	❑	❑	❑	❑
	synphalangism	❑	❑	❑	❑
	not opposition	❑	❑	❑	❑
	proximally placed	❑	❑	❑	❑

specific description of positive findings..
....
....

		RIGHT		LEFT	
		NO	YES	NO	YES
fingers	syndactyly	❑	❑	❑	❑
	synphalangism	❑	❑	❑	❑
	preaxial polydactyly	❑	❑	❑	❑
	postaxial polydactyly	❑	❑	❑	❑
	camptodactyly	❑	❑	❑	❑
	oligodactyly	❑	❑	❑	❑
	adactyly	❑	❑	❑	❑
	clinodactyly V finger	❑	❑	❑	❑
	clinodactyly other fingers	❑	❑	❑	❑
	brachydactyly	❑	❑	❑	❑

arachnodactyly	❑	❑	❑	❑
tapering fingers	❑	❑	❑	❑
broad distal phalanges	❑	❑	❑	❑
normal	❑	❑	❑	❑
metacarpals				
IV shortening	❑	❑	❑	❑
other metacarpal shortening	❑	❑	❑	❑
normal	❑	❑	❑	❑

specific description of positive findings..
....
....

Lower limb

	NO	YES
asymmetry	❑	❑
genu valgus	❑	❑
genu varus	❑	❑
genu recurvatum	❑	❑
knee webbing	❑	❑
hip dislocation	❑	❑
other joint abnormalities	❑	❑

		RIGHT		LEFT	
		NO	YES	NO	YES
shortening	rhizomelic	❑	❑	❑	❑
	mesomelic	❑	❑	❑	❑
	acromelic	❑	❑	❑	❑
femur abnormalities		❑	❑	❑	❑
leg abnormalities		❑	❑	❑	❑

specific description of positive findings..
....
....

		RIGHT		LEFT	
		NO	YES	NO	YES
Foot					
general					
	total length	....		....	
	longitudinal plantar crease	❑	❑	❑	❑
	plantar keratosis	❑	❑	❑	❑
	absent foot	❑	❑	❑	❑
	split foot	❑	❑	❑	❑
	sandal gap	❑	❑	❑	❑
	talipes calcaneovalgus	❑	❑	❑	❑
	metatarsus adductus	❑	❑	❑	❑
	talipes equinovarus	❑	❑	❑	❑
	pes planus	❑	❑	❑	❑
	nail abnormalities	❑	❑	❑	❑
hallux					
	broad	❑	❑	❑	❑
	absent-hypoplastic	❑	❑	❑	❑
	proximally placed	❑	❑	❑	❑

toes

syndactyly II-III	❑	❑	❑	❑
syndactyly other toes	❑	❑	❑	❑
preaxial polydactyly	❑	❑	❑	❑
postaxial polydactyly	❑	❑	❑	❑
overridding toes	❑	❑	❑	❑
oligodactyly	❑	❑	❑	❑
adactyly	❑	❑	❑	❑
brachydactyly	❑	❑	❑	❑
normal	❑	❑	❑	❑

metatarsal

IV shortening	❑	❑	❑	❑
other metatarsal shortening	❑	❑	❑	❑

specific description of positive findings..
....
....

Joints

	NO	YES
hypermobility	❑	❑
dislocations	❑	❑
contractures	❑	❑
enlargement	❑	❑

specific description of positive findings..
....
....

Skin

	NO	YES
hypopigmentation diffuse	❑	❑
hyperpigmentation diffuse	❑	❑
patchy hypopigmentation	❑	❑
café au lait spots	❑	❑
nevi	❑	❑
freckles	❑	❑
teleangiectasias	❑	❑
hemangiomas	❑	❑
easy bruisability	❑	❑
hyperextensibility	❑	❑
dryness	❑	❑
generalized hypertrichosis	❑	❑
generalized hypotrichosis	❑	❑
keratinization abnormalities	❑	❑
normal	❑	❑

specific description of positive findings..
....
....

Neurology

	NO	YES	
mental retardation	❑	❑	
I.Q. done (score and scale)	❑	❑	....

seizures	❑	❑
ataxia	❑	❑

Other neurologic abnormalities...
....
....

X rays and special examinations
Rx skull done   NO ❑   YES ❑..
....
....

Rx mandible   NO ❑   YES ❑...
....
....

Rx cervical spine done   NO ❑   YES ❑..
....
....

Rx spine done   NO ❑ YES ❑...
....
....

Rx hand done   NO ❑   YES ❑..
....
....

Other skeletal Rx ....
....
....

CT inner ear done NO ❑   YES ❑   Michel ❑   Mondini-Alexander ❑   Bing Siebeman ❑
                  Scheibe ❑   Other ❑..

CT middle ear done   NO ❑   YES ❑
                  Malleus: normal ❑ Malformed ❑ Hypoplastic ❑ fused ❑
                  Incus: normal ❑ Malformed ❑ Hypoplastic ❑ fused ❑
                  Stapes: normal ❑ Malformed ❑ Hypoplastic ❑ fused ❑
                  absence of the oval window ❑
                        Other...
....
....

Renal ultrasound examination done   NO ❑   YES ❑   normal ❑   abnormal ❑   ....
....
....

Pyelography done   NO ❑ YES ❑   normal ❑   abnormal ❑..........................

Echocardiography done   NO ❑ YES ❑   Normal ❑   Abnormal ❑...........................

ECG done   NO ❑ YES ❑   normal ❑   QT and rate..
abnormal ❑ ....
....

Specialist ophthalmologic examination done   NO ❑   YES ❑
                        normal ❑   abnormal ❑...
....

Other special examinations...
....
....

Laboratory studies
....
....
....

karyotype...

Table 12.2: Classification of 236 HL patients after a systematic evaluation

Non-syndromic HL Mendelian	76
Non-syndromic HL isolated	46
Non-classified associated findings	43
Syndromic HL Mendelian	41
Environmental*	16
Syndromic HL non-Mendelian	12
Chromosomal	2
Total	236

*includes 8 TORCH complexes

Table 12.3: Syndromic hearing loss

Mendelian			Non-Mendelian	
Waardenburg	type I	6	OAV	9
	type II	4	TORCH	8
Usher type I and II		6	Chromosomal	2
BO/BOR		5	Other	2
Alport X-L		4	CHARGE	1
Treacher Collins		2		
Aural atresia, microtia and conductive HL		2		
Uncommon syndromic HL*		12		
	Total	41	Total	22

* Duane 1; HL+epilepsy 1; TTD 1; Vohwinkel 1; Melkersson 1; Hypochondroplasia 1; Mohr 1; Coffin Siris 1; FAR 1; HL+ myopia 1; Pendred 1; Facioaudiosynphalangism 1.

Table 12.4: Mendelian hearing loss

Autosomal dominant	Non-syndromic	25	
	Syndromic	21	
	Total		46
Autosomal recessive	Non-syndromic	47	
	Syndromic	16	
	Total		63
X-linked	Non-syndromic	1	
	Syndromic	4	
	Total		5
Unclear pattern of inheritance			3
		Total	117

The percentage of specific syndromal diagnosis among the cases of deafness with associated findings is 40%, higher than the expected 15% to 25% in general syndromal diagnosis (we do not have figures for syndromal hearing loss).

The specific syndromic diagnoses are reported in Table 12.3. The specific Mendelian patterns of inheritance in non-syndromal and syndromal HL are reported in Table 12.4: 19% of all the cases examined were recognized to be autosomal dominant, with syndromal and non-syndromal forms almost equally represented (21 versus 25). This high frequency reflects the effectiveness of the familial diagnostic approach.

References

Aase JM (1990) Diagnostic Dysmorphology. New York and London: Plenum.

Buyse ML (1990) Birth Defect Encyclopedia. Dover Mass: Center for Birth Defects Information Services Inc.

Gorlin RJ, Cohen MM, Levin LS (1990) Syndromes of the Head and Neck. Oxford Monographs on Medical Genetics no. 19. Oxford: Oxford University Press.

Gorlin RJ, Toriello HG, Cohen MM (1995) Hereditary Hearing Loss and its Syndromes. Oxford Monographs on Medical Genetics no. 28. Oxford: Oxford University Press.

Hall JG, Froster-Iskenius UG, Allanson JE (1989) Handbook of Normal Physical Measurements. Oxford: Oxford Medical Publications.

Jones KL (1988) Smith's Recognizable Patterns of Human Malformation. Philadelphia, London, Toronto, Montreal, Sydney, Tokyo: WB Saunders Company.

Sensi A, Bettoli V, Calzolari E. Vohwinkel Syndrome (1994) American Journal of Medical Genetics 50: 201–3.

Stevenson RE, Hall JG, Goodman RM (1993) Human Malformations and Related Anomalies. Oxford Monographs on Medical Genetics no. 27. Oxford: Oxford University Press.

Chapter 13
How to collaborate with a molecular genetics laboratory

ANDREW READ

Pedigrees suitable for genetic research

Researchers always want to hear of suitable families for research. If you think you have such families, contact either the laboratory working on the condition for which you feel they are relevant, or your national contact. What is required depends on the stage that research has reached with the family condition. Initial studies use linkage analysis, whereas later stages move towards mutation analysis. In all cases, good clinical descriptions are essential and at least some family members must be willing to donate samples, usually of blood.

How to take a family tree

The key point is to be systematic. Rule lines for the generations on a large sheet of paper. Start with the proband in the centre. Ask systematically about all first, second and third degree relatives, filling in the pedigree as you go. Mark name and maiden name, date of birth, age at death and cause, and relevant medical history. Ask specifically about infant deaths, stillbirths, abortions and consanguinity. Even with a dominant condition, ask about both sides of the family.

Linkage studies

Linkage analysis requires samples from as many family members as possible. It is important to be sure who is affected and who is unaffected.

Autosomal dominant conditions (see Figure 5.1.1)

A minimum for successful analysis would be 10 individuals (affected or unaffected) each of whom has an affected parent. In order of priority samples should be collected from:

* affected people;
* their parents;
* unaffected people who have an affected parent;
* family members who link together people in the pedigree from whom samples have been taken;
* other individuals.

Autosomal recessive conditions (see Figure 5.1.3)

For particular studies, laboratories may set their own criteria for pedigrees to be collected. In general, only families with several affected individuals are useful. The value of a family is greatest when there are many affected cases, when parents of affected people are related (consanguineous marriages), and when affected people are present in more than one branch of the family. Minimum useful families would be:

* three affected children born to unrelated parents;
* two affected children born to consanguineous parents.

Families more than twice this minimum size are particularly valuable for research. Unaffected individuals (apart from parents of affected individuals) are of less value for analysis in recessive conditions than in dominant conditions.

X-linked inheritance (see Figure 5.1.4)

Any family with at least two affected males has some potential for linkage analysis, especially if they have different mothers. Samples should be taken from:

* affected males;
* women with an affected brother *and* an affected son or grandson;
* mothers and unaffected brothers of affected males;
* both parents of carriers.

Offspring of unaffected males, and women with no affected descendants do not usually give useful information for linkage.

Mitochondrial inheritance

Linkage analysis is not useful for mitochondrially inherited conditions.

Mutation analysis

Once the condition has been mapped, smaller families can be useful and the emphasis of genetic research moves towards mutation detection. The priority samples become:

- a sample from a single well-described affected individual, from each separate family;
- with an autosomal dominant condition, if an affected person appears to be the first in the family and unexpectedly has unaffected parents, then samples from that person and those parents are valuable;
- with X-linked conditions, samples from affected males are more valuable than samples from females, even obligate carriers;
- if mitochondrial inheritance is suspected, samples from a single clearly affected individual, and preferably also the person's mother, should be taken. Analysis of mitochondrial mutations is a specialized area, and it is important to discuss plans in advance with the laboratory.

How to collect and send samples

Blood samples for linkage analysis

A venous blood sample, preferably 10 ml, is taken into EDTA, stored at room temperature or 4°C *but not frozen* and despatched to the laboratory to arrive within 48 hours if at all possible.

Blood samples for mutation analysis

For many investigations a sample taken as above is suitable; but a laboratory may request blood for a chromosome analysis or for setting up a cell line. In this case blood, preferably 10 ml, is taken into lithium heparin, kept at room temperature and sent at room temperature to arrive at the laboratory within 48 hours.

Tissues in addition to blood

These are particularly valuable for mitochondrial mutations and the opportunities afforded by biopsies performed during the clinical work-up, for example muscle biopsies, should be borne in mind. Tissue samples should be frozen (–70°C) without fixation.

Part III
Phenotype/genotype
correlation

Chapter 14
Genotypes and phenotypes of non-syndromal hearing impairments

MANUELA MAZZOLI, DAFYDD STEPHENS

Introduction

In the last few years more than 50 loci have been associated with non-syndromal hearing impairment and it has been estimated that about 100 different genes may be responsible for non-syndromal genetic hearing impairment.

At the present time, the question of the relationship between different mutations of a particular gene and the resulting phenotype remain unclear, but should rapidly become clarified in the near future.

The hereditary hearing loss homepage (http://www.uia.ac.be/dnalab/hhh/) (see Chapter 18) plays a vital role in providing updated information on the gene locations, genes and mutations of these genes. However, by its nature it cannot provide all the information necessary for geneticists and audiologists to determine how a family that they have been studying fits into the pattern of genotypes already described.

Much of this information is provided in different ways in the various papers describing the conditions and little effort has been made to present it in a coherent manner. For this to be useful we have sought to produce standardized forms (see Table 14.1), one for each genotype describing the different conditions. These will be incorporated in the HEAR website.

It may be seen from the forms that there are very many gaps, indicating the limits of our information, despite efforts in many cases to contact the original authors. This can only highlight the further work that needs to be done.

We are indebted to our colleagues Geneviève Lina-Granade (Lyon), Valerie Newton (Manchester), Eva Orzan (Padova) and Fei Zhao (Cardiff) for their hard work, which has made this first step possible.

Table 14.1: Non-syndromal hearing-impairment form

Non-Syndromal Hearing Impairment	
Condition:	MIM No:
Autosomal Dominant /Autosomal Recessive /X-linked Dominant/X-linked Recessive/ /Mitochondrial/ Polygenic	
Gene Localization:	Gene Identification:
Mutations identified:	
Geographical location of families:	
Ethnic origins of families: Caucasoid/Negroid/Mongoloid/Other/Unspecified	
Detailed origin of families:	
Hearing Impairment Penetrance: Complete/incomplete/unknown	
Pathology	
Type: Conductive/cochlear/mixed/neural/central	
Severity: Mild/moderate/severe/profound/variable	
Configuration: [1]	
Unilateral/bilateral	
Age of onset: Congenital/birth to 10 years/11 to 30 years/31 to 50 years/over 50 years/variable/uncertain	
Progression: [2]	
Interfamilial variability:	
Tinnitus: Present/absent/variable manifestation/unknown	
Vestibular function: normal/unilateral hypofunction/bilateral hypofunction/unilateral absent/bilateral absent/clinically normal/unknown	
Source References for 1. Gene localization and identification 2. Hearing loss descriptors	
Contributor and address:	Date:
Footnotes: 1. This should include information on its variability. 2. If present define pattern and rate of progression.	

Chapter 15
Phenotype/genotype correlation of autosomal dominant and autosomal recessive non-syndromal hearing impairment

Manuela Mazzoli, Veronica Kennedy,
Valerie Newton, Fei Zhao, Dafydd Stephens

Introduction

Various estimates have been made suggesting between 30 and 100 different genes responsible for non-syndromal autosomal dominant genetic hearing impairment (NSADHI) and a similar number for non-syndromal autosomal recessive impairment (NSARHI). At the time of writing, June 2000, 29 (plus six reserved for publication) gene locations have been found for the former and 26 (plus three reserved) for the latter. Eleven genes have been cloned for NSADHI and seven for NSARHI.

The clinical expressions of these different genotypes have been investigated in an attempt to find clues suggesting the underlying genetic condition. Several difficulties were encountered in correlating clinical expression to its genotype as different genetic conditions may give rise to clinically identical findings and clinical heterogeneity can be seen within the same family. Furthermore, age and/or environmental factors may influence expressivity even in non-progressive conditions and no specific differences can be found in audiograms between genetic and non genetic HI.

Nevertheless, some general information can be derived by comparing AD and AR conditions. In fact, as illustrated in Table 15.1, the AR disorders tend to show complete penetrance, to be congenital and non-progressive, to involve all frequencies and to be severe or profound (Figure 15.1). However, AD conditions have variable penetrance and can be congenital, although the majority have an onset between 11 and 30 years of age, present with progressive hearing impairment and the severity may vary, but tends to be less severe than in AR conditions (Figure 15.2). In a number of cases insufficient information is available (Table 15.2).

79

Table 15.1: Comparison between some AD and AR hearing impairment characteristics described by the authors as phenotypes of related loci. Not all descriptions were thorough and detailed and some have not been described. It is extremely important that geneticists and clinicians collaborate in describing as many details as possible of the clinical presentation.

		AD	AR
Penetrance	Complete	10	11
	Incomplete	5	2
	Unknown	14	13
Range of frequencies	Low	1	/
	Low/mid	1	/
	Low/high	1	/
	Mid	1	
	Mid/high	3	/
	Mid/all	3	/
	High	6	1
	High/all	3	1
	All	5	1
	Not specified	5	23
Onset	Congenital	5	17
	Birth–10	3	1
	11–30	13	/
	31–50	/	/
	Over 50	/	/
	Variable	5	1
	Uncertain	3	7
Progression	Progressive	19	2
	Stable	5	11
	Variable	/	1
	Unspecified	5	12
Tinnitus	Yes	2	/
	No	6	/
	Unknown	20	26
	Variable	1	/
Vestibular function	Normal	12	6
	Absent	2	1
	Hypofunction	2	/
	Unknown	13	19
Interfamilial variability	Yes	7	/
	No	2	2
	Unknown	20	24

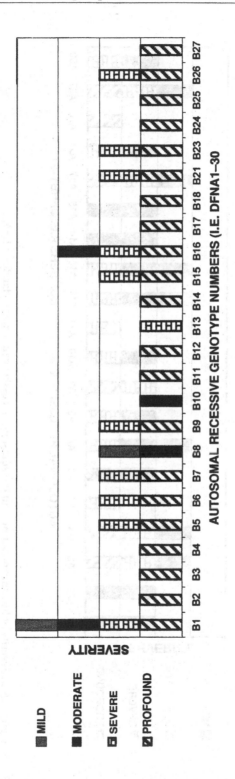

Figure 15.1: Severity of hearing impairment in the autosomal dominant genotypes so far described

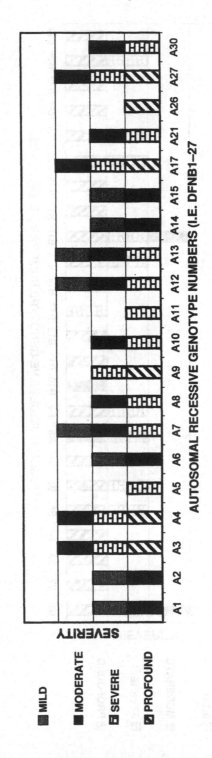

Figure 15.2: Severity of hearing impairment in the autosomal recessive genotypes so far described.

Table 15.2: Cases where insufficient information is available

Hearing Impairment	Autosomal Dominant	Autosomal Recessive
Variable Severity	A20 A23 A24 A25 A28	
Severity Unspecified	A16 A17 A18	B19 B20
Gene Location Reserved	A22 A29 A32 A33 A34 A35	B22 B27 B29
Gene Location Withdrawn	A31	

As mentioned, the majority of genes have not yet been cloned and little is known about the corresponding gene products and their function in the cochlea. The present chapter accounts for the clinical presentation related to the loci associated with hearing impairment. Indeed, it should be emphasized that *loci* represent wide segments of DNA, which may contain one or more abnormal genes and which give no information on the nature of the gene involved or its function. A number of loci may overlap (for example, DFNA17 and DFNB28) or, as has been recently reported, may have a digenic inheritance (for example, the combination of DFNA2 and DFNA12 with the disease alleles on chromosome 1 and 11 is associated with an additive effect resulting in a more severe phenotype than each separately). Another bias can arise from the fact that the phenotype associated with an identified locus derives from the analysis of one or a few families with positive linkage to the locus. Therefore, given the high degree of variability either due to penetrance, ageing or environmental causes that has been observed even within the same family group, it is likely that the phenotypes described will change as more cases are diagnosed with a specific disorder.

As an example of the kind of pitfalls and difficulties that can be encountered in establishing the phenotype of NSHI we can consider the genetic disorders causing a non-syndromal high-frequency hearing impairment.

Coucke et al. (1994) demonstrated linkage to markers on chromosome 1p34 (DFNA2) of a form of non-syndromal, autosomal dominant progressive sensorineural hearing impairment in a large Indonesian family. The hearing impairment first affected the high frequencies during the teens or 20s and became profound within 10 years. Coucke et al. (1994) then performed linkage analyses in an American family and a Dutch family with similar patterns of hereditary hearing impairment. In the Indonesian family, the linkage to 1p was found, whereas in the Dutch family, which had been reported by Huizing et al. (1966), linkage to 1p was excluded. Indeed, there were some clinical differences in the five-generation family studied by Huizing, in which 67 individuals had non-congenital progressive sensorineural HI with onset in early childhood (instead of teens) with impairment at the high frequencies. The impairment increased rapidly with gradual extension to lower frequencies (instead of being slowly progressive across all frequencies). Van Camp et al. (1995) demonstrated, by linkage studies, that the disorder in this family is due to mutation in a gene on 7p15, designated DFNA5. In this cases differences in the clinical presentation could account for different disorders.

Some authors studied the clinical presentation of DFNA2 disorders in details. Marres et al. (1997) examined 43 presumably affected individuals in a six-generation family with DFNA2. Regression analysis showed significant and equi-linear progression of the disorder with age (by about 1 decibel per year) at all frequencies. In 25% to 35% of the patients, an increased vestibulo-ocular reflex was observed (hyper-reactivity) as measured by rotatory responses. These studies should probably be extended to all cases for a better definition of the phenotypes.

Balciuniene et al. (1998) performed linkage studies in a Swedish family with postlingual progressive non-syndromal hearing impairment showing autosomal dominant inheritance. Markers selected for each of two loci, DFNA2 on 1p and DFNA12 on 11q, provided strong indications for linkage, suggesting that both genes contributed to the aetiology of hearing impairment in this family. Further scrutiny of the family showed that severely affected members had haplotypes linked to the disease allele on both chromosomes 1 and 11, whereas individuals with milder hearing loss had haplotypes linked to the disease allele on either chromosome 1 or chromosome 11. The observations suggested an additive effect of two genes, each gene resulting in a mild and sometimes undiagnosed phenotype, but the two together result in a more severe phenotype. This is a possible example of digenic inheritance.

Xia et al. (1998) mapped the gene encoding the connexin GJB3, a protein present in gap junctions in the inner ear, to the DFNA2 region. Mutation analysis revealed that a missense mutation and a nonsense mutation of GJB3 were associated with high-frequency hearing impairment in two Chinese families. Mutations were present also in unaffected family members.

Recently, Kubisch et al. (1999) cloned, in a French family, a second gene to the DNFA2 locus: a new potassium channel protein KCNQ4 present in outer hair cells. Van Hauwe et al. (1999) suggest the possibility of the presence of a third gene causing hearing impairment in this region. Therefore a locus may contain more than one gene specifically involved in hearing function and each gene may have several mutations which may account for differences in clinical presentation.

Another location, DFNA3 (13q11-12), may give rise to high to all-frequency hearing impairment with pre-lingual onset, stable or progressive, mild to profound and with incomplete penetrance.

Kelsell et al. (1997) studied a pedigree containing individuals with autosomal dominant deafness and have identified a mutation in the gene encoding the gap-junction protein connexin 26 (Cx26 or GJB2). Cx26 mutations resulting in premature stop codons were also found in three autosomal recessive non-syndromal sensorineuronal hearing impairment pedigrees with profound, fully penetrant, prelingual hearing impairment, genetically linked to chromosome 13q11-12 (DFNB1), where the Cx26 gene is localized. Several mutations of Cx26 have been identified.

DFNA7 (1q21-23) may also give rise to high-frequency, progressive, mild-to-severe hearing impairment, with onset between 11 and 30 years of age and incomplete penetrance. Several candidate genes have been considered for this location (Fagerheim et al., 1996).

The genes responsible for non-syndromal hearing impairment are likely to have specific roles in the hearing process. Little is known at the molecular level about the process of hearing in the cochlea, and virtually nothing is known about the genes involved.

In the future, as research will lead to cloning of genes and to the identification of related products, it will probably shed some light on the relationship between the clinical presentation and the site and/or function of gene anomalies in the inner ear as well as the influence of age and environmental factors.

The clinical presentation can be useful in discriminating between different genetic conditions, especially if several parameters are considered as well as the audiogram. Nevertheless it cannot be consider specific. We suggest the following tables in which several parameters are considered (Table 15.3) as standard for the definition of the phenotypes.

It may be seen from the forms that there are very many gaps, indicating the limits of our information, despite efforts in many cases to contact the original authors. This can only highlight the further work that needs to be done.

Acknowledgements

We are indebted to our colleagues Geneviève Lina-Granade (Lyon), Valerie Newton (Manchester), Eva Orzan (Padova) and Fei Zhao (Cardiff) for their hard work, which has made this first step possible.

Table 15.3: Completed non-syndromal hearing impairment forms

Non-Syndromal Hearing Impairment	
Condition: DFNA1	**MIM No:** 124900
Autosomal Dominant	
Gene Localization: 5q31	**Gene Identification:** Homologue of Drosophila diaphanous (HD1A1)
Mutations identified: Protein truncating mutation caused by a single nucleotide substitution	
Penetrance: Complete	
Pathology: Regulation of polymerization of actin re hair cell cytoskeleton	
Geographical location of families: Costa Rica	
Ethnic origins of families: Hispanic	
Detailed origin of families: Unspecified	
Hearing Impairment	
Type: Cochlear	
Severity: Mild – Severe	
Configuration: Low-frequency hearing impairment	
Bilateral	
Age of onset: 11 to 30 years	
Progression: Progressive (slowly through adolescence)	
Interfamilial variability: Unknown	
Tinnitus: Present	
Vestibular function: Normal	
Source References for **1. Gene localization & identification** • *Leon et al (1992) Proc Natl Acad Sc 189:5181-5184* • *Lynch et al (1997) Science 278:1315-1318* **2. Hearing Impairment descriptors** • *Leon et al (1981) Am J Hum Genet 33:209-214*	
Contributors & address: Fei Zhao,Dafydd Stephens,Veronica Kennedy Welsh Hearing Institute, Cardiff, Wales	**Date:** 21/12/99

Non-Syndromal Hearing Impairment	
Condition: DFNA2	**MIM No:** 600101
Autosomal Dominant	
Gene Localization: 1p34	**Gene Identification:** KCNQ4 + Connexin 31(GJB3)
Mutations identified: missense/nonsense mutations of GJB3, missense/deletion mutations of KCNQ4	
Penetrance: Unknown	
Pathology: Affects sensory outer hair cells	
Geographical location of families: Indonesia, USA, Netherlands, Belgium, China	
Ethnic origins of families: Unspecified	
Detailed origin of families: Indonesia, France, Luxemburg, Netherlands, Belgium,China	
Hearing Impairment **Type:** Cochlear	
Severity: Mild – Severe	
Configuration: High-frequency hearing impairment → all frequencies	
Bilateral	
Age of onset: 11 to 30 years in Indonesian families, others may be <10	
Progression: Progressive (Profound within 10 years of onset)	
Interfamilial variability: Present	
Tinnitus: Variable manifestation, may be the initial symptom	
Vestibular function: Normal	
Source References for **1. Gene localization & identification** • *Van Camp et al (1997) Geonomics 41:70-74* • *Kubisch et al (1999) Cell 96:437-46* **2. Hearing Impairment descriptors** • *Coucke et al (1994) New Eng J Med 331:425-431* • *Xia et al (1998) Nat Genet 20:370-3*	
Contributors & address: Fei Zhao,Dafydd Stephens,Veronica Kennedy Welsh Hearing Institute, Cardiff, Wales	**Date:** 21/12/99

Non-Syndromal Hearing Impairment	
Condition: DFNA3	**MIM No:** 601544
Autosomal Dominant	
Gene Localization: 13q12	**Gene Identification:** Connexin 26 (GJB2 +GJB6)
Mutations identified: M34T	
Penetrance: Incomplete	
Pathology: Unknown	
Geographical location of families: France, Not specified	
Ethnic origins of families: Unspecified	
Detailed origin of families: France, Not specified	
Hearing Impairment	
Type: Cochlear	
Severity: Moderate – Profound	
Configuration: High to all frequencies hearing impairment	
Bilateral	
Age of onset: Congenital	
Progression: Stable	
Interfamilial variability: Unknown	
Tinnitus: Unknown	
Vestibular function: Normal	
Source References for	
1. Gene localization & identification	
• *Kelsell et al (1997) Nature 387:80-83*	
• *Grifa et al (1999) Nat Genet 23:16-18*	
2. Hearing Impairment descriptors	
• *Chaib et al (1994) Hum Molec Genet 3:2219-22*	
• *Kelsell et al (1997) Nature 387:80-83*	
Contributors & address: Fei Zhao and Dafydd Stephens Welsh Hearing Institute, Cardiff, Wales	**Date:** 3/4/98

Non-Syndromal Hearing Impairment	
Condition: DFNA4	**MIM No:** 600652
Autosomal Dominant	
Gene Localization: 19q13	**Gene Identification:** Unknown
Mutations identified: Unknown	
Penetrance: Unknown	
Pathology: Unknown	
Geographical location of families: USA	
Ethnic origins of families: Unspecified	
Detailed origin of families: Unspecified	
Hearing Impairment **Type:** Cochlear	
Severity: Moderate – Profound	
Configuration: All frequency hearing impairment	
Bilateral	
Age of onset: 11 to 30 years	
Progression: Progressive (severe-Profound by 4th decade)	
Interfamilial variability: Unknown	
Tinnitus: Unknown	
Vestibular function: Unknown	

Source References for
 	
1. Gene localization & identification
 	
  • *Chen et al (1995) Hum Molec Genet 4:1073-76*
 	
2. Hearing Impairment descriptors
 	
  • *Chen et al (1995) Hum Molec Genet 4:1073-76*	

Contributors & address: Fei Zhao and Dafydd Stephens Welsh Hearing Institute, Cardiff, Wales	**Date:** 3/4/98

Non-Syndromal Hearing Impairment	
Condition: DFNA5	**MIM No:** 600994
Autosomal Dominant	
Gene Localization: 7p15	**Gene Identification:** DFNA5
Mutations identified: Premature truncation, deletion mutation	
Penetrance: Complete	
Pathology: Unknown	
Geographical location of families: Netherlands	
Ethnic origins of families: Caucasoid	
Detailed origin of families: Dutch	
Hearing Impairment **Type:** Cochlear	
Severity: Severe	
Configuration: High-frequency hearing impairment	
Bilateral	
Age of onset: 11 to 30 years	
Progression: Progressive (rapidly in first 3 decades)	
Interfamilial variability: Unknown	
Tinnitus: Unknown	
Vestibular function: Normal	

Source References for
 	
 1. Gene localization & identification
 	
    • *Van Camp et al (1995) Hum Mol Genet 4:2159-2163*
 	
    • *Van Camp et al (1998) Am J Hum Genet 63 Suppl A52*
 	
 2. Hearing Impairment descriptors
 	
    • *Huizing et al (1966) Acta Otolaryngol 61, 35-41: 161-167*
 	
    • *Huizing et al (1983) Acta Otolayngol 95: 620-626*	

Contributors & address: Dafydd Stephens, Veronica Kennedy Welsh Hearing Institute, Cardiff, Wales	**Date:** 21/12/99

Non-Syndromal Hearing Impairment	
Condition: DFNA6	MIM No: 600965
Autosomal Dominant	
Gene Localization: 4p16.3	Gene Identification: Unknown
Mutations identified: Unknown	
Penetrance: Incomplete	
Pathology: Unknown	
Geographical location of families: USA	
Ethnic origins of families: Unspecified	
Detailed origin of families: Unspecified	
Hearing Impairment	
Type: Cochlear	
Severity: Mild – Moderate	
Configuration: Low- and high-frequency hearing impairment - "Hill-type" pattern in 1st decade with mid-frequencies later affected	
Bilateral	
Age of onset: 11 to 30 years	
Progression: Progressive, but may stabilize	
Interfamilial variability: Present	
Tinnitus: Absent	
Vestibular function: Normal	
Source References for	
1. Gene localization & identification	
• *Lesperance et al (1995) Hum Molec Genet 4:1967-72*	
2. Hearing Impairment descriptors	
• *The Vanderbilt University Hereditary Deafness Study Group (1968) Arch Otolaryngol 88:242-50*	
Contributor & address: Dafydd Stephens, Veronica Kennedy Welsh Hearing Institute, Cardiff, Wales	Date: 21/12/99

Non-Syndromal Hearing Impairment	
Condition: DFNA7	**MIM No:** 601412
Autosomal Dominant	
Gene Localization: 1q21-23	**Gene Identification:** Unknown
Mutations identified: Unknown	
Penetrance: Incomplete	
Pathology: Unknown	
Geographical location of families: Norway	
Ethnic origins of families: Caucasoid	
Detailed origin of families: Norwegian	
Hearing Impairment	
Type: Cochlear	
Severity: Mild–Severe	
Configuration: High-frequency hearing impairment	
Bilateral	
Age of onset: 11 to 30 years	
Progression: Progressive (approaching a gently sloping pattern in mid-life)	
Interfamilial variability: Present	
Tinnitus: Unknown	
Vestibular function: Normal	
Source References for	
1. Gene localization & identification	
• *Fagerheim et al (1996) Hum Molec Genet 5:1187-91*	
2. Hearing Impairment descriptors	
• *Fagerheim et al (1996) Hum Molec Genet 5:1187-91*	
Contributors & address: Fei Zhao and Dafydd Stephens Welsh Hearing Institute, Cardiff, Wales	**Date:** 3/4/98

Non-Syndromal Hearing Impairment	
Condition: DFNA8 (See also DFNA12)	**MIM No:** 601543
Autosomal Dominant	
Gene Localization: 11q22-24	**Gene Identification:** TECTA
Mutations identified: missense mutation	
Penetrance: Unknown	
Pathology: Tectorial membrane defect	
Geographical location of families: Austria	
Ethnic origins of families: Caucasoid	
Detailed origin of families: Unspecified	
Hearing Impairment	
Type: Cochlear	
Severity: Moderate–Severe	
Configuration: All frequencies: U-shaped form with maximal loss at 2 kHz	
Bilateral	
Age of onset: Congenital/birth to 10 years	
Progression: Stable	
Interfamilial variability: None	
Tinnitus: Unknown	
Vestibular function: Normal	
Source References for	
1. Gene localization & identification	
• *Verhoeven et al (1998) Nat Genet 19:60-2*	
• *Kirschhofer et al (1996) Cytogenet Cell Genet 82(1-2)126-30*	
2. Hearing Impairment descriptors	
• *Kirschhofer et al (1996) Cytogenet Cell Genet 82(1-2)126-30*	
Contributor & address: Fei Zhao, Dafydd Stephens,Veronica Kennedy Welsh Hearing Institute Cardiff, Wales	**Date:** 21/12/99

Non-Syndromal Hearing Impairment	
Condition: DFNA9	**MIM No:** 601394
Autosomal Dominant	
Gene Localization: 14q12-q13	**Gene Identification:** COCH
Mutations identified: 3 missense mutations	
Penetrance: Complete	
Pathology: Mucoplysaccharide deposits in neural channels of osseous spiral lamina and vestibular labyrinth	
Geographical location of families: USA, Netherlands, Belgium	
Ethnic origins of families: Unspecified	
Detailed origin of families: Unspecified	
Hearing Impairment **Type:** Sensorineural	
Severity: Severe / Profound	
Configuration: High – all frequencies	
Bilateral	
Age of onset: 11 to 30 years	
Progression: Progressive (Profound in mid-life)	
Interfamilial variability: Present	
Tinnitus: Absent	
Vestibular function: Abnormal	

Source References for
 	
1. Gene localization & identification
 	
  • *Manolis et al (1996) Hum Molec Genet 5:1047-1050*
 	
  • *Robertson et al (1998) Nature Genetics 20:299-303*
 	
2. Hearing Impairment descriptors
 	
  • *Khetarpal et al (1991) Arch Otolaryngol 117: 1032-1042*
 	
  • *De Kok et al (1999) Hum Molec Genet 8: 361-6*	

Contributors & address: Fei Zhao, Dafydd Stephens, Veronica Kennedy Welsh Hearing Institute, Cardiff, Wales	**Date:** 21/12/99

Non-Syndromal Hearing Impairment	
Condition: DFNA10	**MIM No:** 601316
Autosomal Dominant	
Gene Localization: 6q22-23	**Gene Identification:** Unknown
Mutations identified: Unknown	
Penetrance: Complete	
Pathology: Unknown	
Geographical location of families: USA	
Ethnic origins of families: Unspecified	
Detailed origin of families: Unspecified	
Hearing Impairment	
Type: Cochlear	
Severity: Moderate–Severe	
Configuration: All frequencies	
Bilateral	
Age of onset: Variable	
Progression: Progressive	
Interfamilial variability: Unknown	
Tinnitus: Unknown	
Vestibular function: Unknown	
Source References for	
1. Gene localization & identification	
• *O Neil et al. (1996) Hum Molec Genet 5:853-6*	
2. Hearing Impairment descriptors	
• *O Neil et al. (1996) Hum Molec Genet 5:853-6*	
Contributors & address: Fei Zhao and Dafydd Stephens Welsh Hearing Institute, Cardiff, Wales	**Date:** 3/4/98

Non-Syndromal Hearing Impairment	
Condition: DFNA11	**MIM No:** 601317
Autosomal Dominant	
Gene Localization: 11q12.3-q21	**Gene Identification:** MYO7A
Mutations identified: 9-bp deletion of exon 22	
Penetrance: Complete	
Pathology: Unknown	
Geographical location of families: Japan, China	
Ethnic origins of families: Unspecified	
Detailed origin of families: Japan, China	
Hearing Impairment **Type:** Cochlear	
Severity: Severe	
Configuration: High-frequency hearing impairment	
Bilateral	
Age of onset: Variable	
Progression: Progressive	
Interfamilial variability: Unknown	
Tinnitus: Unknown	
Vestibular function: Bilaterally absent	
Source References for **1. Gene localization & identification** • *Tamagawa et al. (1996) Hum Molec Genet 5:849-852* • *Liu et al. (1997) Nature Genet 17:268-9* **2. Hearing Impairment descriptors** • *Tamagawa et al. (1996) Hum Molec Genet 5:849-852* • *Liu et al. (1997) Nature Genet 17:268-9*	
Contributors & address: Fei Zhao,Dafydd Stephens,Veronica Kennedy Welsh Hearing Institute, Cardiff, Wales	**Date:** 12/12/99

Non-Syndromal Hearing Impairment	
Condition: DFNA12 (See also DFNA8)	**MIM No:** 601842
Autosomal Dominant	
Gene Localization: 11q22-24	**Gene Identification:** TECTA
Mutations identified: missense mutations	
Penetrance: Complete	
Pathology: affects tectorial membrane	
Geographical location of families: Belgium, Austria	
Ethnic origins of families: Unspecified	
Detailed origin of families: Belgium, Austria	
Hearing Impairment **Type:** Cochlear	
Severity: Mild–Severe	
Configuration: Mid-frequency hearing impairment	
Bilateral	
Age of onset: Congenital/Birth to 10 years	
Progression: Stable	
Interfamilial variability: Unknown	
Tinnitus: Unknown	
Vestibular function: Normal	
Source References for **1. Gene localization & identification** • *Verhoeven et al. (1997) Am J Hum Genet 60:1168-73* • *Verhoeven et al. (1998) Nat Genet 19:60-2* **2. Hearing Impairment descriptors** • *Verhoeven et al. (1997) Am J Hum Genet 60:1168-73*	
Contributors & address: Fei Zhao,Dafydd Stephens,Veronica Kennedy Welsh Hearing Institute, Cardiff, Wales	**Date:** 21/12/99

Non-Syndromal Hearing Impairment	
Condition: DFNA13	**MIM No:** 601868
Autosomal Dominant	
Gene Localization: 6p21.3	**Gene Identification:** COL11A2
Mutations identified: Unknown	
Penetrance: Unknown	
Pathology: Unknown	
Geographical location of families: USA, Netherlands	
Ethnic origins of families: Unspecified	
Detailed origin of families: Unspecified	
Hearing Impairment	
Type: Cochlear	
Severity: Mild/Severe	
Configuration: Mid-frequency hearing impairment in childhood, across all frequencies in adult	
Bilateral	
Age of onset: 11 to 30 years	
Progression: Progressive	
Interfamilial variability: Unknown	
Tinnitus: Absent	
Vestibular function: Normal	
Source References for	
1. Gene localization & identification	
• *McGuirt et al (1999) Nat Genet 23:413-9*	
• *Van Camp et al (1997) Am J Hum Genet 60:758-64*	
2. Hearing Impairment descriptors	
• *Kunst et al (2000) Am J Otol, 21:181-7*	
• *Brown et al (1997) Am J Genet 61:924-27*	
Contributors & address: Fei Zhao,Dafydd Stephens,Veronica Kennedy Welsh Hearing Institute, Cardiff, Wales	**Date:** 21/12/99

Non-Syndromal Hearing Impairment	
Condition: DFNA14	**MIM No:**
Autosomal Dominant	
Gene Localization: 4p16.3	**Gene Identification:** Unknown
Mutations identified: Unknown	
Penetrance: Incomplete	
Pathology: Unknown	
Geographical location of families: USA, Netherlands	
Ethnic origins of families: Unspecified	
Detailed origin of families: Unspecified	
Hearing Impairment	
Type: Cochlear	
Severity: Mild/Moderate	
Configuration: Low- + Mid-frequency hearing impairment especially at 2kHz	
Bilateral	
Age of onset: 11 to 30 years	
Progression: Progressive	
Interfamilial variability: Present	
Tinnitus: Absent	
Vestibular function: Usually normal	
Source References for	
1. Gene localization & identification	
• *Van Camp et al. (1999) J Med Genet 36:532-6*	
2. Hearing Impairment descriptors	
• *Kunst et al (1999) Audiology 38:165-173*	
• *Van Camp et al. (1999) J Med Genet 36:532-6*	
Contributors & address: Dafydd Stephens and Veronica Kennedy Welsh Hearing Institute, Cardiff, Wales	**Date:** 21/12/99

Non-Syndromal Hearing Impairment	
Condition: DFNA15	**MIM No:** 602459 602460
Autosomal Dominant	
Gene Localization: 5q31	**Gene Identification:** POU4F3
Mutations identified: Eight base pair deletion	
Penetrance: Complete	
Pathology: Unknown	
Geographical location of families: Israel	
Ethnic origins of families: Jewish	
Detailed origin of families: North Africa, Israel	
Hearing Impairment **Type:** Sensorineural	
Severity: Moderate/Severe	
Configuration: All frequencies	
Bilateral	
Age of onset: 11 to 30 years	
Progression: Progressive	
Interfamilial variability: Unknown	
Tinnitus: No	
Vestibular function: Abnormal	

Source References for
 	
1. Gene localization & identification
 	
  • *Vahava et al (1998) Science 279:1950-1954*
 	
2. Hearing Impairment descriptors
 	
  • *Vahava et al (1998) Science 279:1950-1954*
 	
  • *Frydman et al (2000) Arch Otolaryngol Head Neck Surg 126:633-7*	

Contributors & address: Dafydd Stephens and Veronica Kennedy Welsh Hearing Institute, Cardiff, Wales	**Date:** 03/06/00

Non-Syndromal Hearing Impairment	
Condition: DFNA16	**MIM No:** 603964
Autosomal Dominant	
Gene Localization: 2q23-24.3	**Gene Identification:** Unknown
Mutations identified: Unknown	
Penetrance: Unknown	
Pathology: Unknown	
Geographical location of families: Unspecified	
Ethnic origins of families: Unspecified	
Detailed origin of families: Unspecified	
Hearing Impairment	
Type: Sensorineural	
Severity: Unspecified	
Configuration: Sloping high-frequency fluctuating hearing impairment responsive to steroids	
Bilateral	
Age of onset: 11 to 30 years	
Progression: Progressive	
Interfamilial variability: Present	
Tinnitus: Present	
Vestibular function: Unknown	
Source References for	
1. Gene localization & identification	
• *Fukushiwa et al (1999) Am J Hum Genet 65:141-50*	
2. Hearing Impairment descriptors	
• *Fukushiwa et al (1999) Am J Hum Genet 65:141-50*	
Contributors & address: Dafydd Stephens and Veronica Kennedy Welsh hearing Institute, Cardiff, Wales	**Date:** 21/12/99

Non-Syndromal Hearing Impairment	
Condition: DFNA17 (Overlaps DFNB28)	**MIM No:** 603622
Autosomal Dominant	
Gene Localization: 22q12.2-13.3	**Gene Identification:** Unknown
Mutations identified: Unknown	
Penetrance: Complete	
Pathology: Cochleosaccular degeneration with degeneration of the Organ of Corti, saccular epithelium and stria vascularis. Also loss of neurones and gliosis in inferior olivary nucleus.	
Geographical location of families: USA	
Ethnic origins of families: Unspecified	
Detailed origin of families: Unspecified	
Hearing Impairment **Type:** Cochlear / Neural	
Severity: Moderate / Profound	
Configuration: High-frequency initially to severe hearing impairment by 3rd decade across all frequencies	
Bilateral	
Age of onset: 4 to 10 years	
Progression: Progressive	
Interfamilial variability: Present	
Tinnitus: Unknown	
Vestibular function: Unknown	

Source References for
 	
1. Gene localization & identification
 	
   • *Lalwani et al (1999)Am J Hum Genet 64:318-23*
 	
2. Hearing Impairment descriptors
 	
   • *Lalwani et al (1999)Am J Hum Genet 64:318-23*	

Contributors & address: Dafydd Stephens and Veronica Kennedy Welsh hearing Institute, Cardiff, Wales	**Date:** 21/12/99

Non-Syndromal Hearing Impairment	
Condition: DFNA18	**MIM No:**
Autosomal Dominant	
Gene Localization: 3q22	**Gene Identification:** Unknown
Mutations identified: Unknown	
Penetrance: Unknown	
Pathology: Unknown	
Geographical location of families: Germany	
Ethnic origins of families: Unspecified	
Detailed origin of families: Unspecified	
Hearing Impairment	
Type: Unspecified	
Severity: Unspecified	
Configuration: Unspecified	
Unilateral/bilateral: Unspecified	
Age of onset: Uncertain	
Progression: Unspecified	
Interfamilial variability: Unknown	
Tinnitus: Unknown	
Vestibular function: Unknown	
Source References for	
1. Gene localization & identification	
• *Boensch et al (1998) Am J Hum Genet 63 Suppl A282*	
2. Hearing Impairment descriptors	
Contributor & address: Dafydd Stephens Welsh hearing Institute, Cardiff, Wales	**Date:** 8/12/98

Non-Syndromal Hearing Impairment	
Condition: DFNA19	**MIM No:**
Autosomal Dominant	
Gene Localization:10 pericentromic	**Gene Identification:** Unknown
Mutations identified: Unknown	
Penetrance: Unknown	
Pathology: Unknown	
Geographical location of families: Unspecified	
Ethnic origins of families: Unspecified	
Detailed origin of families: Unspecified	
Hearing Impairment **Type:** Unknown	
Severity: Unspecified	
Configuration: Unspecified	
Unilateral/bilateral: Unspecified	
Age of onset: Uncertain	
Progression: Unspecified	
Interfamilial variability: Unknown	
Tinnitus: Unknown	
Vestibular function: Unknown	
Source References for **1. Gene localization & identification** • *Green et al (1998) Human Biol Hearing & Deafness, Bethesda Oct 8-11 1998 Abstract 107* **2. Hearing Impairment descriptors**	
Contributor & address: Dafydd Stephens Welsh hearing Institute, Cardiff, Wales	**Date:** 8/12/98

Non-Syndromal Hearing Impairment	
Condition: DFNA20 (Overlaps with DFNA26)	**MIM No:**
Autosomal Dominant	
Gene Localization: 17q25	**Gene Identification:** Unknown
Mutations identified: Unknown	
Penetrance: Complete	
Pathology: Unknown	
Geographical location of families: USA	
Ethnic origins of families: Caucasoid	
Detailed origin of families: English	
Hearing Impairment **Type:** Cochlear / Sensorineural	
Severity: Variable	
Configuration: Sloping high-frequency hearing impairment, first evident at 6 + 8 kHz	
Bilateral	
Age of onset: 11 to 30 years	
Progression: Progressive	
Interfamilial variability: Unknown	
Tinnitus: Unknown	
Vestibular function: Normal	

Source References for
 1. Gene localization & identification
   • *Morell et al (2000) Geonomics 63:1-6*
 2. Hearing Impairment descriptors
   • *Morell et al (2000) Geonomics 63:1-6*	

Contributors & address: Dafydd Stephens and Veronica Kennedy Welsh Hearing Institute, Cardiff, Wales	**Date:** 12/03/00

Non-Syndromal Hearing Impairment	
Condition: DFNA21	**MIM No:**
Autosomal Dominant	
Gene Localization: 6p21-22	**Gene Identification:** Unknown
Mutations identified: Unknown	
Penetrance: Incomplete	
Pathology: Unknown	
Geographical location of families: Netherlands	
Ethnic origins of families: Unspecified	
Detailed origin of families: Dutch	
Hearing Impairment	
Type: Unspecified	
Severity: Moderate/Severe	
Configuration: Mid-frequency / Flattened to downsloping	
Bilateral	
Age of onset: Pre- + post-lingual, up to 45y	
Progression: Progressive	
Interfamilial variability: Unknown	
Tinnitus: None	
Vestibular function: Normal	
Source References for **1. Gene localization & identification** • *Kunst et al (2000) Clin Otolaryngol 25:45-54* **2. Hearing Impairment descriptors** • *Kunst et al (2000) Clin Otolaryngol 25:45-54*	
Contributors & address: Veronica Kennedy Welsh Hearing Institute, Cardiff, Wales	**Date:** 21/01/2000

Non-Syndromal Hearing Impairment	
Condition: DFNA23	**MIM No:**
Autosomal Dominant	
Gene Localization: 14q21-q22	**Gene Identification:** Unknown
Mutations identified: Unknown	
Penetrance: Complete	
Pathology: Unknown	
Geographical location of families: Switzerland	
Ethnic origins of families: Caucasoid	
Detailed origin of families: German	
Hearing Impairment	
Type: Cochlear / Mixed	
Severity: Variable	
Configuration: Hearing impairment mild at low frequencies, variable at mid frequencies, moderate to profound at high frequencies. Conductive component in 50% of cases.	
Bilateral	
Age of onset: Congenital / <1 year old	
Progression: Stable	
Interfamilial variability: Unknown	
Tinnitus: Unknown	
Vestibular function: Unknown	
Source References for	
1. Gene localization & identification	
• *Salam et al (2000) Am J Hum Genet 66:1984-1988*	
2. Hearing Impairment descriptors	
• *Salam et al (2000) Am J Hum Genet 66(6)):1984-1988*	
Contributor & address: Veronica Kennedy Welsh Hearing Institute, Cardiff, Wales	**Date:** 03/06/00

Non-Syndromal Hearing Impairment	
Condition: DFNA24	**MIM No:**
Autosomal Dominant	
Gene Localization: 4q35-qter	**Gene Identification:** Unknown
Mutations identified: Unknown	
Penetrance: Unknown	
Pathology: Unknown	
Geographical location of families: Switzerland	
Ethnic origins of families: Caucasoid	
Detailed origin of families: German	
Hearing Impairment **Type:** Sensorineural	
Severity: Variable	
Configuration: Sloping hearing impairment in the mid – high frequencies	
Bilateral	
Age of onset: Prelingual	
Progression: Stable	
Interfamilial variability: Unknown	
Tinnitus: Unknown	
Vestibular function: Unknown	

Source References for
 	
1. Gene localization & identification
 	
    • *Hafner et al (2000) Am J Hum Genet 66:1437-1442*
 	
2. Hearing Impairment descriptors
 	
    • *Hafner et al (2000) Am J Hum Genet 66:1437-1442*	

Contributor & address: Veronica Kennedy Welsh Hearing Institute, Cardiff, Wales	**Date:** 06/05/00

Non-Syndromal Hearing Impairment	
Condition: DFNA25	**MIM No:**
Autosomal Dominant	
Gene Localization: 12q21-24	**Gene Identification:** Unknown
Mutations identified: Unknown	
Penetrance: Unknown	
Pathology: Unknown	
Geographical location of families: USA	
Ethnic origins of families: Unspecified	
Detailed origin of families: Czech	
Hearing Impairment	
Type: Sensorineural	
Severity: Variable	
Configuration: High frequency hearing impairment	
Bilateral	
Age of onset: 11 to 30 years	
Progression: Progressive	
Interfamilial variability: Unknown	
Tinnitus: Unknown	
Vestibular function: Unknown	
Source References for	
1. Gene localization & identification	
• *Greene et al (1999) American Society of Human Genetics Meeting , San Francisco, Oct 19-23 1999 Prog Nr 1399*	
2. Hearing Impairment descriptors	
• *Greene et al (1999) American Society of Human Genetics Meeting , San Francisco, Oct 19-23 1999 Prog Nr 1399*	
Contributor & address: Veronica Kennedy Welsh Hearing Institute, Cardiff, Wales	**Date:** 21/12/99

Non-Syndromal Hearing Impairment	
Condition: DFNA26 (Overlaps with DFNA20)	**MIM No:**
Autosomal Dominant	
Gene Localization: 17q25	**Gene Identification:** Unknown
Mutations identified: Unknown	
Penetrance: Unknown	
Pathology: Unknown	
Geographical location of families: USA	
Ethnic origins of families: AngloEuropean	
Detailed origin of families: Unspecified	
Hearing Impairment	
Type: Sensorineural	
Severity: Profound	
Configuration: Unspecified	
Bilateral	
Age of onset: Congenital	
Progression: Unspecified	
Interfamilial variability: Unknown	
Tinnitus: Unknown	
Vestibular function: Unknown	
Source References for **1. Gene localization & identification** • *Smith, R - unpublished* **2. Hearing Impairment descriptors**	
Contributor & address: Veronica Kennedy Welsh Hearing Institute, Cardiff, Wales	**Date:** 21/12/99

Non-Syndromal Hearing Impairment	
Condition: DFNA27	**MIM No:**
Autosomal Dominant	
Gene Localization: 4q12	**Gene Identification:** Unknown
Mutations identified: Unknown	
Penetrance: Unknown	
Pathology: Unknown	
Geographical location of families: USA	
Ethnic origins of families: Unspecified	
Detailed origin of families: Unspecified	
Hearing Impairment **Type:** Sensorineural	
Severity: Moderate / Profound	
Configuration: Unspecified	
Bilateral	
Age of onset: Pre-teens – late 20s	
Progression: Unspecified	
Interfamilial variability: Unknown	
Tinnitus: Unknown	
Vestibular function: Unknown	
Source References for **1. Gene localization & identification** • *Fridell et al (1999) American Society of Human Genetics Meeting, San Francisco, Oct 19-23 1999 Prog Nr 1388* **2. Hearing Impairment descriptors** • *Fridell et al (1999) American Society of Human Genetics Meeting, San Francisco, Oct 19-23 1999 Prog Nr 1388*	
Contributor & address: Veronica Kennedy Welsh Hearing Institute, Cardiff, Wales	**Date:** 21/12/99

Non-Syndromal Hearing Impairment	
Condition: DFNA28	MIM No:
Autosomal Dominant	
Gene Localization: 8q22	Gene Identification: Unknown
Mutations identified: Unknown	
Penetrance: Unknown	
Pathology: Unknown	
Geographical location of families: USA	
Ethnic origins of families: Unspecified	
Detailed origin of families: Unspecified	
Hearing Impairment Type: Cochlear	
Severity: Variable	
Configuration: Mid – high frequency hearing impairment	
Bilateral	
Age of onset: >7 years	
Progression: Progressive	
Interfamilial variability: Unknown	
Tinnitus: Unknown	
Vestibular function: Unknown	

Source References for
 	
 1. Gene localization & identification
 	
    • *Anderson et al (1999) American Society of Human Genetics Meeting, San Francisco,*
 	
      Oct 19-23 1999 Prog Nr 1336
 	
 2. Hearing Impairment descriptors
 	
    • *Anderson et al (1999) American Society of Human Genetics Meeting, San Francisco,*
 	
      Oct 19-23 1999 Prog Nr 1336	

Contributor & address: Veronica Kennedy Welsh Hearing Institute, Cardiff, Wales	Date: 21/12/99

Non-Syndromal Hearing Impairment	
Condition: DFNA30	**MIM No:**
Autosomal Dominant	
Gene Localization: 15q26	**Gene Identification:** Unknown
Mutations identified: Unknown	
Penetrance: Unknown	
Pathology: Unknown	
Geographical location of families: Veneto Region (Italy)	
Ethnic origins of families: Caucasoid	
Detailed origin of families: Italian	
Hearing Impairment **Type:** Cochlear	
Severity: Moderate – Severe	
Configuration: Mid- to high-frequency hearing impairment	
Bilateral	
Age of onset: Birth to 10 years	
Progression: Progressive until 4th decade then stable	
Interfamilial variability: No	
Tinnitus: No	
Vestibular function: Hypofunction	
Source References for **1. Gene localization & identification** • *Mangino et al (1999) American Society of Human Genetics Meeting, San Francisco,* *Oct 19-23 1999 Prog Nr 2459* **2. Hearing Impairment descriptors** • *Mangino et al (1999) American Society of Human Genetics Meeting, San Francisco,* *Oct 19-23 1999 Prog Nr 2459*	
Contributor & address: Veronica Kennedy Welsh Hearing Institute, Cardiff, Wales Manuela Mazoli, Audiologia, University of Ferrara	**Date:** 30/5/00

Non-Syndromal Hearing Impairment	
Condition: DFNA36	**MIM No:**
Autosomal Dominant	
Gene Localization: 9q13 -q21	**Gene Identification:** Unknown
Mutations identified: Unknown	
Penetrance: Unknown	
Pathology: Unknown	
Geographical location of families: Not specified	
Ethnic origins of families: Not specified	
Detailed origin of families: Not specified	
Hearing Impairment **Type:** Not specified	
Severity: Not specified	
Configuration: Not specified	
Unilateral/Bilateral: Not specified	
Age of onset: Not specified	
Progression: Not specified	
Interfamilial variability: Not specified	
Tinnitus: Not specified	
Vestibular function: Not specified	
Source References for **1. Gene localization & identification** • *Van Camp G, Smith RJH. Hereditary Hearing Loss Homepage. (update 15/6/00)* *http://dnalab-www.uia.ac.be/dnalab/hhh/* **3. Hearing Impairment descriptors**	
Contributor & address: Veronica Kennedy Welsh Hearing Institute, Cardiff, Wales	**Date:** 16/6/00

Non-Syndromal Hearing Impairment	
Condition: DFNB1	**MIM No:** 220290
Autosomal Recessive	
Gene Localization: 13q11-12	**Gene Identification:** Connexin 26 (GJB2)
Mutations identified: Missense, Stopcodons, Deletion, Nonsense mutations	
Penetrance: Complete	
Pathology: Affects stria vascularis, basement membranes, limbus, spiral prominence	
Geographical location of families: Tunisia, France, New Zealand, Australia, Britain, Italy, Spain, Pakistan	
Ethnic origins of families: Caucasoid	
Detailed origin of families: Anglo-Celtic in Australia/New Zealand	
Hearing Impairment	
Type: Cochlear	
Severity: Mild – Profound	
Configuration: Flat – high frequency sloping	
Bilateral	
Age of onset: Congenital	
Progression: Stable	
Interfamilial variability: Unknown	
Tinnitus: Unknown	
Vestibular function: Unknown	
Source References for	
1. Gene localization & identification	
• *Guilford et al (1994a) Nature Genetics 6: 24 - 28*	
• *Kelsell et al (1997) Nature Genetics 387: 80 - 83*	
2. Hearing impairment descriptors	
• *Maw et al (1995) Am J Hum Genet 57: 629 – 35*	
• *Denoyelle et al (1999) Lancet 353: 1298 - 303*	
Contributors & addresses: Valerie Newton, University of Manchester Veronica Kennedy, Welsh Hearing Institute	**Date:** 21/12/99

Non-Syndromal Hearing Impairment	
Condition: DFNB2	**MIM No:** 600060
Autosomal Recessive	
Gene Localization: 11q13-14	**Gene Identification:** MYO7A
Mutations identified: Arg 244 Pro substitution, T insertion mutation, G to A transition in exon 15	
Penetrance: Complete	
Pathology: Affects IHC & OHC – mainly IHC – Region of stereocilia	
Geographical location of families: Tunisia, S. India, Lebanon, China	
Ethnic origins of families: Caucasoid / Mongoloid	
Detailed origin of families: Unspecified	
Hearing Impairment **Type:** Cochlear	
Severity: Profound	
Configuration: Unspecified	
Bilateral	
Age of onset: 0 to 16 years	
Progression: Stable	
Interfamilial variability: None	
Tinnitus: Unknown	
Vestibular function: Bilateral hypofunction / Bilaterally absent	

Source References for
 	
 1. Gene localization & identification
 	
  • *Guilford et al (1994b) Hum Mol Genet 3: 989- 93*
 	
  • *Liu et al (1997) Nature Genetics 16: 188 – 190*
 	
 2. Hearing impairment descriptors
 	
  • *Liu et al (1997) Nature Genetics 16: 188 – 190*	

Contributors & addresses: Valerie Newton, University of Manchester Veronica Kennedy, Welsh Hearing Institute	**Date:** 21/12/99

Non-Syndromal Hearing Impairment	
Condition: DFNB3	**MIM No:** 600316
Autosomal Recessive	
Gene Localization: 17p11.2 – q 12	**Gene Identification:** MYO15
Mutations identified: 2 missense mutations, 1 nonsense mutation	
Penetrance: Unknown	
Pathology: Unknown	
Geographical location of families: Bali, India	
Ethnic origins of families: Caucasoid	
Detailed origin of families: Unspecified	
Hearing Impairment	
Type: Cochlear	
Severity: Profound	
Configuration: Unspecified	
Bilateral	
Age of onset: Congenital	
Progression: Stable	
Interfamilial variability: None	
Tinnitus: Unknown	
Vestibular function: Clinically normal	
Source References for	
1. Gene localization & identification	
• *Friedman et al (1995) Nature Genetics 9: 86 - 91*	
• *Wang et al (1998) Science 280:1447-51*	
2. Hearing impairment descriptiors	
Contributors & addresses: Valerie Newton, University of Manchester Veronica Kennedy, Welsh Hearing Institute	**Date:** 21/12/99

Non-Syndromal Hearing Impairment	
Condition: DFNB4	**MIM No:** 600791
Autosomal Recessive Syndromal – Pendred S.	
Gene Localization: 7q 31	**Gene Identification:** PDS
Mutations identified: missense mutation in PDS	
Penetrance: Incomplete	
Pathology: enlarged vestibular aqueduct	
Geographical location of families: Israel, Japan	
Ethnic origins of families: Caucasoid, Mongoloid	
Detailed origin of families: Druze in Israel	
Hearing Impairment	
Type: Cochlear	
Severity: Profound (>70dB)	
Configuration: High frequency	
Bilateral	
Age of onset: Congenital	
Progression: Stable, fluctuating, sometimes progressive	
Interfamilial variability: Unknown	
Tinnitus: Unknown	
Vestibular function: Unknown	
Source References for	
1. Gene localization & identification	
• *Baldwin et al (1995) Hum Mol Genet 4: 1637 - 1642*	
• *Usami et al (1999) Hum Genet 104: 188-92*	
2. Hearing impairment descriptors	
• *Usami et al (1999) Hum Genet 104: 188-92*	
Contributors & addresses: Valerie Newton University of Manchester Veronica Kennedy Welsh Hearing Institute	**Date:** 21/12/99

Non-Syndromal Hearing Impairment	
Condition: DFNB5 (Originally reported as DFNB4)	**MIM No:** 600792
Autosomal Recessive	
Gene Localization: 14q12	**Gene Identification:** Unknown
Mutations identified: Unknown	
Penetrance: Complete	
Pathology: Unknown	
Geographical location of families: USA and India	
Ethnic origins of families: Caucasoid	
Detailed origin of families: Unspecified	
Hearing Impairment	
Type: Cochlear	
Severity: Severe / Profound	
Configuration: Unspecified	
Bilateral	
Age of onset: Congenital	
Progression: Stable	
Interfamilial variability: Unknown	
Tinnitus: Unknown	
Vestibular function: Unknown	
Source References for	
1. Gene localization & identification	
• *Fukushima et al (1995a) Hum Mol Genet 4: 1643 - 1648*	
2. Hearing impairment descriptors	
Contributor & address: Valerie Newton The University of Manchester	**Date:** 3/4/98

Non-Syndromal Hearing Impairment	
Condition: DFNB6	**MIM No:** 600971
Autosomal Recessive	
Gene Localization: 3p 14 - 21	**Gene Identification:** Unknown
Mutations identified: Unknown	
Penetrance: Complete	
Pathology: Unknown	
Geographical location of families: USA, India	
Ethnic origins of families: Caucasoid	
Detailed origin of families: Unspecified	
Hearing Impairment **Type:** Cochlear	
Severity: Severe / Profound	
Configuration: Unspecified	
Bilateral	
Age of onset: Congenital	
Progression: Stable	
Interfamilial variability: Unknown	
Tinnitus: Unknown	
Vestibular function: Unknown	
Source References for **1. Gene localization & identification** • *Fukushima et al (1995) Genome Research 5: 305 - 308* **2. Hearing impairment descriptors**	
Contributor & address: Valerie Newton University of Manchester	**Date:** 3/4/98

Non-Syndromal Hearing Impairment	
Condition: DFNB7	**MIM No:** 600974
Autosomal Recessive	
Gene Localization: 9q 13 - 21	**Gene Identification:** Unknown
Mutations identified: Unknown	
Penetrance: Complete	
Pathology: Unknown	
Geographical location of families: India	
Ethnic origins of families: Caucasoid	
Detailed origin of families: Unspecified	
Hearing Impairment	
Type: Cochlear	
Severity: Severe / Profound	
Configuration: Unspecified	
Bilateral	
Age of onset: Congenital	
Progression: Stable	
Interfamilial variability: Unknown	
Tinnitus: Unknown	
Vestibular function: Unknown	
Source References for	
1. Gene localization & identification	
• *Jain et al (1995) Hum Mol Genet 4: 2391 - 2394*	
2. Hearing impairment descriptors	
Contributor & address: Valerie Newton University of Manchester	**Date:** 3/4/98

Non-Syndromal Hearing Impairment	
Condition: DFNB8	**MIM No:** 601072
Autosomal Recessive	
Gene Localization: 21q22	**Gene Identification:** Unknown
Mutations identified: Unknown	
Penetrance: Unknown	
Pathology: Unknown	
Geographical location of families: Pakistan	
Ethnic origins of families: Caucasoid	
Detailed origin of families: Unspecified	
Hearing Impairment **Type:** Cochlear	
Severity: Moderate / Severe	
Configuration: Unspecified	
Bilateral	
Age of onset: 10 to 12 years	
Progression: Progressive	
Interfamilial variability: Unknown	
Tinnitus: Unknown	
Vestibular function: Unknown	
Source References for **1. Gene localization & identification** • *Veske et al (1996) Hum Mol Genet 5: 165 - 168* **2. Hearing impairment descriptors**	
Contributor & address: Valerie Newton University of Manchester	**Date:** 3/4/98

Non-Syndromal Hearing Impairment	
Condition: DFNB9 (Originally reported as DFNB6)	**MIM No:** 601071
Autosomal Recessive	
Gene Localization: 2p 22-23	**Gene Identification:** OTOF
Mutations identified: nonsense mutation Y730X	
Penetrance: Complete	
Pathology: affects cochlear IHC and vestibular type I sensory hair cells	
Geographical location of families: Lebanon, Eastern Turkey	
Ethnic origins of families: Caucasoid	
Detailed origin of families: Sunni	
Hearing Impairment **Type:** Cochlear	
Severity: Severe/profound	
Configuration: Unspecified	
Bilateral	
Age of onset: Congenital	
Progression: Stable	
Interfamilial variability: Unknown	
Tinnitus: Unknown	
Vestibular function: Clinically normal	
Source References for **1. Gene localization & identification** • *Chaib et al (1996a) Hum Mol Genet 5: 155 - 158* • *Yasunaga et al (1999) Nat Genet 21: 363 - 9* **2. Hearing impairment descriptors**	
Contributors & addresses: Valerie Newton University of Manchester Veronica Kennedy Welsh Hearing Institute	 **Date:** 21/12/99

Non-Syndromal Hearing Impairment	
Condition: DFNB10	**MIM No:** 601386
Autosomal Recessive	
Gene Localization: 21q22.3	**Gene Identification:** TMPRSS3
Mutations identified: Unknown	
Penetrance: Complete	
Pathology: Unknown	
Geographical location of families: Palestine	
Ethnic origins of families: Caucasoid	
Detailed origin of families: Unspecified	
Hearing Impairment **Type:** Cochlear	
Severity: Severe (> 75 – 80 dB)	
Configuration: Unspecified	
Bilateral	
Age of onset: Congenital	
Progression: Stable	
Interfamilial variability: Unknown	
Tinnitus: Unknown	
Vestibular function: Clinically normal	
Source References for **1. Gene localization & identification** • *Bonne-Tamiv et al (1996) Am J. Hum Genet 58: 1254 - 1259* • *Wattenhofer et al (2000) Europ.Soc.Hum.Genet (Abstract)* **2. Hearing impairment descriptors**	
Contributor & address: Valerie Newton University of Manchester Veronica Kennedy Welsh Hearing Institute	**Date:** 15/6/00

Non-Syndromal Hearing Impairment	
Condition: DFNB11	**MIM No:**
Autosomal Recessive	
Gene Localization: 9q13 - q21	**Gene Identification:** Unknown
Mutations identified: Unknown	
Penetrance: Unknown	
Pathology: Unknown	
Geographical location of families: Middle East, Israel	
Ethnic origins of families: Caucasoid	
Detailed origin of families: Bedouin	
Hearing Impairment	
Type: Cochlear	
Severity: Profound	
Configuration: Unspecified	
Bilateral	
Age of onset: Congenital	
Progression: Stable	
Interfamilial variability: Unknown	
Tinnitus: Unknown	
Vestibular function: Unknown	
Source References for	
1. Gene localization & identification	
• *Scott et al (1996) AM J. Hum Genet 59: 389 - 391*	
2. Hearing impairment descriptors	
Contributor & address: Valerie Newton University of Manchester	**Date:** 3/4/98

Non-Syndromal Hearing Impairment	
Condition: DFNB12	**MIM No:** 601386
Autosomal Recessive	
Gene Localization: 10q 21-22	**Gene Identification:** Unknown
Mutations identified: Unknown	
Penetrance: Complete	
Pathology: Unknown	
Geographical location of families: Syria	
Ethnic origins of families: Caucasoid	
Detailed origin of families: Sunni	
Hearing Impairment **Type:** Cochlear	
Severity: Profound	
Configuration: Unspecified	
Bilateral	
Age of onset: Congenital	
Progression: Stable	
Interfamilial variability: Unknown	
Tinnitus: Unknown	
Vestibular function: Unknown	
Source References for **1. Gene localization & identification** • *Chaib et al (1966b) Hum Mol Genet 5: 1061 - 1064* **2. Hearing impairment descriptors**	
Contributor & address: Valerie Newton University of Manchester	**Date:** 3/4/98

Non-Syndromal Hearing Impairment	
Condition: DFNB13	**MIM No:** 603098
Autosomal Recessive	
Gene Localization: 7q 34-36	**Gene Identification:** Unknown
Mutations identified: Unknown	
Penetrance: Unknown	
Pathology: Unknown	
Geographical location of families: Lebanon	
Ethnic origins of families: Caucasoid	
Detailed origin of families: Unspecified	
Hearing Impairment	
Type: Sensorineural / Central	
Severity: Severe	
Configuration: Unspecified	
Unilateral/bilateral: Unspecified	
Age of onset: Uncertain	
Progression: Progressive	
Interfamilial variability: Unknown	
Tinnitus: Unknown	
Vestibular function: Unknown	
Source References for	
1. Gene localization & identification	
• *Mustapha et al (1998) Eur J. Hum Gen 6: 245 - 50*	
2. Hearing impairment descriptors	
Contributors & addresses: Valerie Newton University of Manchester Veronica Kennedy Welsh Hearing Institute	**Date:** 21/12/99

Non-Syndromal Hearing Impairment	
Condition: DFNB14	**MIM No:** 603098
Autosomal Recessive	
Gene Localization: 7q31	**Gene Identification:** Unknown
Mutations identified: Unknown	
Penetrance: Unknown	
Pathology: Unknown	
Geographical location of families: Lebanon	
Ethnic origins of families: Caucasoid	
Detailed origin of families: Unspecified	
Hearing Impairment **Type:** Neural / Central	
Severity: Profound	
Configuration: Unknown	
Unilateral/bilateral: Unspecified	
Age of onset: Congenital / Birth to 10 years (pre-lingual)	
Progression: Unknown	
Interfamilial variability: Unknown	
Tinnitus: Unknown	
Vestibular function: Unknown	
Source References for **1. Gene localization & identification** • *Mustapha et al 1998 Eur J Hum Genet 6: 548 - 51* **2. Hearing impairment descriptors**	
Contributors & addresses: Valerie Newton University of Manchester Veronica Kennedy Welsh Hearing Institute	**Date:** 21/12/99

Non-Syndromal Hearing Impairment	
Condition: DFNB15	**MIM No:** 601869
Autosomal Recessive	
Gene Localization: 3q21-q25 on 19p13	**Gene Identification:** Unknown
Mutations identified: Unknown	
Penetrance: Complete	
Pathology: Unknown	
Geographical location of families: India	
Ethnic origins of families: Caucasoid	
Detailed origin of families: Unspecified	
Hearing Impairment	
Type: Cochlear	
Severity: Severe / Profound	
Configuration: Unspecified	
Bilateral	
Age of onset: Prelingual	
Progression: Stable	
Interfamilial variability: Unknown	
Tinnitus: Unknown	
Vestibular function: Clinically normal	
Source References for	
1. Gene localization & identification	
• *Chen et al (1997) Am J. Med Gen 71: 467 - 471*	
2. Hearing impairment descriptors	
Contributor & address: Valerie Newton University of Manchester	**Date:** 3/4/98

Non-Syndromal Hearing Impairment	
Condition: DFNB16	**MIM No:** 603720
Autosomal Recessive	
Gene Localization: 15q 21 - q 22	**Gene Identification:** Unknown
Mutations identified: Unknown	
Penetrance: Complete	
Pathology: Unknown	
Geographical location of families: Pakistan, Middle East	
Ethnic origins of families: Caucasoid	
Detailed origin of families: Unspecified	
Hearing Impairment **Type:** Cochlear	
Severity: Moderate / Profound	
Configuration: Unknown	
Bilateral	
Age of onset: Congenital	
Progression: Unknown	
Interfamilial variability: Unknown	
Tinnitus: Unknown	
Vestibular function: Unknown	
Source References for **1. Gene localization & identification** • *Campbell et al (1997) J. Med Genet 34: 1015 - 1017* **2. Hearing impairment descriptors**	
Contributors & addresses: Valerie Newton University of Manchester Veronica Kennedy Welsh Hearing Institute	**Date:** 21/12/99

Non-Syndromal Hearing Impairment	
Condition: DFNB17	**MIM No:** 603010
Autosomal Recessive	
Gene Localization: 7q 31	**Gene Identification:** Unknown
Mutations identified: Unknown	
Penetrance: Unknown	
Pathology: Unknown	
Geographical location of families: Madras, Southern India	
Ethnic origins of families: Caucasoid	
Detailed origin of families: Tamil	
Hearing Impairment	
Type: Sensorineural	
Severity: Profound	
Configuration: all frequencies	
Bilateral	
Age of onset: Congenital	
Progression: Unknown	
Interfamilial variability: Unspecified	
Tinnitus: Unknown	
Vestibular function: Normal	
Source References for	
1. Gene localization & identification	
• *Greinwald et al, AM. J. Med Gen 78: 107 - 13*	
2. Hearing impairment descriptors	
• *Greinwald et al, AM. J. Med Gen 78: 107 – 13*	
Contributors & addresses: Valerie Newton University of Manchester Veronica Kennedy Welsh Hearing Institute	**Date:** 21/12/99

Non-Syndromal Hearing Impairment	
Condition: DFNB18	**MIM No:** 602092
Autosomal Recessive	
Gene Localization: 11p14 - 15.1	**Gene Identification:** Unknown
Mutations identified: Unknown	
Penetrance: Complete	
Pathology: Unknown	
Geographical location of families: India	
Ethnic origins of families: Caucasoid	
Detailed origin of families: Unspecified	
Hearing Impairment	
Type: Cochlear	
Severity: Profound	
Configuration: Unspecified	
Bilateral	
Age of onset: Congenital	
Progression: Unknown	
Interfamilial variability: Unknown	
Tinnitus: Unknown	
Vestibular function: Normal	
Source References for	
1. Gene localization & identification	
• *Jain et al (1998) Genomics 50: 290 - 2*	
2. Hearing impairment descriptors	
Contributors & addresses: Valerie Newton University of Manchester Veronica Kennedy Welsh Hearing Institute	**Date:** 21/12/99

Non-Syndromal Hearing Impairment	
Condition: DFNB19	**MIM No:**
Autosomal Recessive	
Gene Localization: 18p11	**Gene Identification:** Unknown
Mutations identified: Unknown	
Penetrance: Unknown	
Pathology: Unknown	
Geographical location of families: Unspecified	
Ethnic origins of families: Unspecified	
Detailed origin of families: Unspecified	
Hearing Impairment	
Type: Unspecified	
Severity: Unspecified	
Configuration: Unspecified	
Unilateral/bilateral: Unspecified	
Age of onset: Uncertain	
Progression: Unspecified	
Interfamilial variability: Unspecified	
Tinnitus: Unknown	
Vestibular function: Unknown	
Source References for	
1. Gene localization & identification	
• *Green et al (1998) Human Biol Hearing & Deafness, Bethesda Oct 8-11 1998 Abstract 1072.*	
2. Hearing impairment descriptors	
Contributors & addresses: Valerie Newton University of Manchester Veronica Kennedy Welsh Hearing Institute	 **Date:** 21/12/99

Non-Syndromal Hearing Impairment	
Condition: DFNB20	**MIM No:** 604060
Autosomal Recessive	
Gene Localization: 11q25-qter	**Gene Identification:** Unknown
Mutations identified: Unknown	
Penetrance: Unknown	
Pathology: Unknown	
Geographical location of families: Pakistan	
Ethnic origins of families: Caucasoid	
Detailed origin of families: Unspecified	
Hearing Impairment	
Type: Unspecified	
Severity: Unspecified	
Configuration: Unspecified	
Unilateral/bilateral: Unspecified	
Age of onset: Uncertain	
Progression: Unspecified	
Interfamilial variability: Unspecified	
Tinnitus: Unknown	
Vestibular function: Unknown	
Source References for	
1. Gene localization & identification	
• *Moynihan et al 1999 Eur J Hum Genet 7: 243 - 6*	
2. Hearing impairment descriptors	
Contributors & addresses: Valerie Newton University of Manchester Veronica Kennedy Welsh Hearing Institute	**Date:** 21/12/99

Non-Syndromal Hearing Impairment	
Condition: DFNB21	**MIM No:** 603629
Autosomal Recessive	
Gene Localization: 11q23-25	**Gene Identification:** TECTA
Mutations identified: G to A transition in the donor splice site (GT) of intron 9	
Penetrance: Unknown	
Pathology: Unknown	
Geographical location of families: Lebanon	
Ethnic origins of families: Caucasoid	
Detailed origin of families: Unspecified	
Hearing Impairment	
Type: Neural / Central	
Severity: Severe / Profound	
Configuration: Unspecified	
Unilateral/bilateral: Unspecified	
Age of onset: Congenital / Birth to 10 years (pre-lingual)	
Progression: Unspecified	
Interfamilial variability: Unknown	
Tinnitus: Unknown	
Vestibular function: Unknown	
Source References for	
1. Gene localization & identification	
• *Mustapha et al (1999) Hum Mol Genet 8: 409 - 12*	
2. Hearing impairment descriptors	
• *Mustapha et al (1999) Hum Mol Genet 8: 409 - 12*	
Contributor & address: Veronica Kennedy, Welsh Hearing Institute, Cardiff, Wales	**Date:** 21/12/99

Non-Syndromal Hearing Impairment	
Condition: DFNB23	**MIM No:**
Autosomal Recessive	
Gene Localization: 10p11.2 - q21	**Gene Identification:** Unknown
Mutations identified: Unknown	
Penetrance: Unknown	
Pathology: Unknown	
Geographical location of families: Unspecified	
Ethnic origins of families: Indian	
Detailed origin of families: Unspecified	
Hearing Impairment **Type:** Sensorineural	
Severity: Severe / Profound	
Configuration: Unknown	
Bilateral	
Age of onset: Uncertain	
Progression: Unspecified	
Interfamilial variability: Unspecified	
Tinnitus: Unknown	
Vestibular function: Unknown	
Source References for **1. Gene localization & identification** • *Richard Smith, unpublished* **2. Hearing impairment descriptors**	
Contributor & address: Veronica Kennedy, Welsh Hearing Institute, Cardiff, Wales	**Date:** 21/12/99

Non-Syndromal Hearing Impairment	
Condition: DFNB24	**MIM No:**
Autosomal Recessive	
Gene Localization: 11q23	**Gene Identification:** Unknown
Mutations identified: Unknown	
Penetrance: Unknown	
Pathology: Unknown	
Geographical location of families: Unspecified	
Ethnic origins of families: Indian	
Detailed origin of families: Unspecified	
Hearing Impairment	
Type: Unspecified	
Severity: Profound	
Configuration: Unspecified	
Bilateral	
Age of onset: Uncertain	
Progression: Unspecified	
Interfamilial variability: Unspecified	
Tinnitus: Unknown	
Vestibular function: Unknown	
Source References for	
1. Gene localization & identification	
• *Richard Smith, unpublished*	
2. Hearing impairment descriptors	
Contributor & address: Veronica Kennedy, Welsh Hearing Institute, Cardiff, Wales	**Date:** 21/12/99

Non-Syndromal Hearing Impairment	
Condition: DFNB25	**MIM No**
Autosomal Recessive	
Gene Localization: 4p15.3 - q12	**Gene Identification:** Unknown
Mutations identified: Unknown	
Penetrance: Unknown	
Pathology: Unknown	
Geographical location of families: Unspecified	
Ethnic origins of families: Indian	
Detailed origin of families: Unspecified	
Hearing Impairment	
Type: Unspecified	
Severity: Profound	
Configuration: Unspecified	
Bilateral	
Age of onset: Uncertain	
Progression: Unspecified	
Interfamilial variability: Unspecified	
Tinnitus: Unknown	
Vestibular function: Unknown	
Source References for **1. Gene localization & identification** • *Richard Smith, unpublished* **2. Hearing impairment descriptors**	
Contributor & address: Veronica Kennedy, Welsh Hearing Institute, Cardiff, Wales	**Date:** 21/12/99

Non-Syndromal Hearing Impairment	
Condition: DFNB26	**MIM No:**
Autosomal Recessive	
Gene Localization: (4q2 modif. 1q22-23) 4q28	**Gene Identification:** Unknown
Mutations identified: Unknown	
Penetrance: Incomplete	
Pathology: Unknown	
Geographical location of families: Pakistan	
Ethnic origins of families: Caucasoid	
Detailed origin of families: Unspecified	
Hearing Impairment	
Type: Unspecified	
Severity: Severe / Profound	
Configuration: Unspecified	
Unilateral/bilateral: Unspecified	
Age of onset: Uncertain	
Progression: Unspecified	
Interfamilial variability: Unspecified	
Tinnitus: Unknown	
Vestibular function: Unknown	
Source References for **1. Gene localization & identification** • *Riazzuddin et al 1999 Abstract from American Society of Human Genetics Meeting in San Francisco Oct 19 - 23 1999 Program Nr.530* **2. Hearing impairment descriptors**	
Contributor & address: Veronica Kennedy, Welsh Hearing Institute, Cardiff, Wales	**Date:** 21/12/99

Non-Syndromal Hearing Impairment	
Condition: DFNB28	**MIM No:**
Autosomal Recessive	
Gene Localization: 22q13	**Gene Identification:**
Mutations identified:	
Penetrance: Unknown	
Pathology: Unknown	
Geographical location of families: Palestine	
Ethnic origins of families: Caucasoid: Jewish + Palestinian	
Detailed origin of families: Unspecified	
Hearing Impairment	
Type: Neural / Central	
Severity: Profound	
Configuration: Unspecified	
Bilateral	
Age of onset: Congenital	
Progression: Unspecified	
Interfamilial variability: Unspecified	
Tinnitus: Unknown	
Vestibular function: Unknown	
Source References for	
1. Gene localization & identification	
• *Kanaan et al (1999) Abstract from American Society of Human Genetics Meeting in San Francisco Oct 19 - 23 1999 Program Nr: 1703*	
2. Hearing impairment descriptors	
Contributor & address: Veronica Kennedy, Welsh Hearing Institute, Cardiff, Wales	**Date:** 21/12/99

References

Balciuniene J, Dahl N, Borg E, Samuelsson E, Koisti MJ, Pettersson U, Jazin EE (1998) Evidence for digenic inheritance of non-syndromic hereditary hearing loss in a Swedish family. American Journal of Human Genetics 63: 786–93.

Coucke P, Van Camp G, Djoydiharjo B, Smith SD, Frants RR, Padberg GW, Darby JK, Huizing EH, Cremers CWRJ, Kimberling WJ, Oostra BA, Van de Heyning PH, Willems PJ, (1994) Linkage of autosomal dominant hearing loss to the short arm of chromosome 1 in two families. New England Journal of Medicine 331: 425–31.

Fagerheim T, Nilssen O, Raeymaekers P, Brox V, Moum T, Elverland HH, Teig E, Omland HH, Fostad GK, Tranebjaerg (1996) Identification of a new locus for autosomal dominant non-syndromic hearing impairment (DFNA7) in large Norwegian family. Human Molecular Genetics Aug 5(8): 1187–91.

Huizing EH, Van Bolhuis AH, Odenthal DW (1966) Studies on progressive hereditary perceptive deafness in a family of 335 members. I. Genetical and general audiological results. Acta Otolaryngologia 61: 35–41.

Kelsell DP, Dunlop J, Stevens HP, Lench NJ, Liang JN, Parry G, Mueller RF, Leigh IM (1997) Connexin 26 mutations in hereditary non-syndromic sensorineural deafness. Nature May 1, 387(6628): 80–3.

Kubisch C, Schroeder BC, Friedrich T, Lutjohann B, El-Amraoui A, Marlin S, Petit C, Jentsch TJ (1999) KCNQ4, a novel potassium channel expressed in sensory outer hair cells, is mutated in dominant deafness. Cell 96: 437–46.

Marres H, van Ewijk M, Huygen P, Kunst H, van Camp G, Coucke P, Willems P, Cremers C (1997) Inherited non-syndromic hearing loss: an audiovestibular study in a large family with autosomal dominant progressive hearing loss related to DFNA2. Archives in Otolaryngology and Head and Neck Surgery 123: 573–77.

Van Camp G, Coucke P, Balemans W, Van Velzen D, Van de Bilt C, Van Laer L, Smith RJH, Fukushima K, Padberg GW, Frants RR, Van de Heyning P, Smith SD, Huizing EH, Willems PJ (1995) Localization of a gene for non-syndromic hearing loss (DFNA5) to chromosome 7p15. Human Molecular Genetics 4: 2159–63.

Van Hauwe P, Coucke PJ, Declau F, Kunst H, Ensink RJ, Marres HA, Cremers CWRJ, Djelantik B, Smith SD, Kelley P, Van de Heyning PH, Van Camp G (1999) Deafness linked to DFNA2: one locus but how many genes? (Letter) Nature Genetics 21: 263 only.

Xia J, Liu C, Tang B, Pan Q, Huang L, Dai H, Zhang B, Xie W, Hu D, Zheng D, Shi X, Wang D, Xia K, Yu K, Liao X, Feng Y, Yang Y, Xiao J, Xie D, Huang J (1998) Mutations in the gene encoding gap junction protein beta-3 associated with autosomal dominant hearing impairment. Nature Genetics 20: 370–73.

Chapter 16
Genotypes and phenotypes of non-syndromal X-linked hearing impairment

Manuela Mazzoli, Eva Orzan, Dafydd Stephens

Introduction

Non-syndromal X-linked hearing impairment is a rare form of genetic hearing impairment, accounting for a small proportion of all hereditary hearing impairment. It is both clinically and genetically heterogeneous and five loci have been described to date but only two of these have been mapped. One is pending (reserved) although not yet published.

The difficulties encountered in the analysis of autosomal dominant (AD), recessive (AR) and mitochondrial disorders associated with hearing impairment are found also for X-linked conditions associated with impairment of the hearing function. In fact, the *loci* represent wide segments of DNA, which may contain one or more abnormal genes and give no information on the nature of the gene involved or its function and different mutations or anomalies can give rise to quite diverse phenotypes. This is well illustrated by the history of research about *DFN1*.

In 1960, a large Norwegian family was described in which males in four generations were affected by an early-onset progressive form of sensorineural impairment (Mohr and Mageroy, 1960), which was indexed in McKusick as *DFN1*. Sufficient hearing was present at first for speech to develop normally, but then it deteriorated. Impaired hearing first became apparent at age 3 to 5 years. No associated symptoms were described at that time. A later study of the original *DFN1* family showed that the hearing impairment is part of a progressive X-linked recessive syndrome, which includes visual impairment, dystonia, fractures and mental deficiency. Some obligate carrier females showed signs of minor neuropathy and mild hearing impairment (Tranebjaerg et al., 1995). Therefore, *DFN1* is a syndromal form of deafness (Mohr and Tranebjaerg syndrome) and does not actually belong in the list of non-syndromal forms of hearing impairment.

Linkage analysis localized the locus involved to a region in Xq22 closely linked to the COL4A5 gene, the site of the mutation in X-linked Alport syndrome. However, there was no family history of renal disease. This can give an idea of how minute the alterations can be and that close regions may control very different functions.

Further analysis, using positional information from a patient with a 21-kb deletion in Xq22 and sensorineural hearing impairment together with dystonia, Jin et al. (1996) characterized a novel transcript lying within the deletion as a candidate gene for the complex syndrome of Mohr and Tranebjaerg (MTS). They discovered small deletions in this candidate gene in the original Norwegian family and in a family with hearing impairment, dystonia, and mental deficiency but not blindness. This gene, which they named DDP (deafness/dystonia peptide), showed high levels of expression in foetal and adult brains. Thus it is likely that the DDP gene encodes an evolutionarily conserved novel polypeptide necessary for normal human neurological development. The three families in which Jin et al. (1996) demonstrated mutations in the DDP gene displayed overlapping but not identical hearing impairment phenotypes. The disease was most severe in the original Norwegian family, where mental deterioration and blindness were evident in virtually every affected individual, and least severe in the patient and his affected relatives who suffered only from hearing impairment and dystonia and showed a 21-kb deletion in Xq22. The mental deterioration and blindness associated with the MTS phenotype typically occurred later in life, and no affected male in the large deletion family had survived beyond the age of nine years due to the higher morbidity associated with having X-linked agammaglobulinemia. One patient (Vetric et al., 1993) had been found to have a deletion of the BTK gene that extended into a second gene, designated DXS1274E, lying 3-prime of BTK. This was the gene that was subsequently renamed DDP by Jin et al. (1996). The DDP gene lies at the centromeric end of a cluster of five transcripts, three of which, GLA, BTK, and DDP, are known to be involved in genetic disorders. To complicate the picture of DFN1 further, the Mohr-Tranebjaerg syndrome has features that overlap those of Jensen syndrome of opticoacoustic nerve atrophy with dementia and the ataxia-dementia syndrome. Indeed, Tranebjaerg et al. (1997) demonstrated other alterations in the DFN1 gene: a nonsense mutation in a male patient with Jensen syndrome and a TGA insertion in the non-coding region of the DFN1 gene in a male with isolated dystonia.

Koehler et al. (1999) identified the function of the DDP gene, which is mutant in the Mohr-Tranebjaerg syndrome. They demonstrated that DDP is similar to five small mitochondrial proteins of the yeast mitochondrial intermembrane space that mediate the import of metabolite transporters from the cytoplasm into the mitochondrial inner membrane.

Furthermore, another X-linked condition associated with congenital profound sensorineural hearing impairment is linked to Xq22. Tyson et al. (1996) described a four-generation family with this phenotype in which female carriers have a mild/moderate hearing loss affecting the high frequencies. This condition appears to be non-syndromal.

The association of X-linked mixed hearing impairment with stapes gusher has been recognized for 20 years. In the DFN3 condition, mapped to Xq21.1, males present with severe progressive mixed hearing impairment and absent or markedly reduced vestibular responses; obligate female carriers range from normal hearing to a moderate hearing impairment (Cremers and Huygen, 1983). None of the obligate female carriers showed vestibular abnormalities such as those observed in the affected males. DFN3 patients have radiological anomalies of the lateral end of the internal acoustic canal. Phelps et al. (1991) concluded that this results in a communication between the subarachnoid space in the internal auditory meatus and the perilymph in the cochlea, leading to perilymphatic hydrops and a 'gusher' if the stapes is disturbed.

De Kok et al. (1995) demonstrated that the defect in DFN3 resides in a transcription factor with a POU domain known as brain-4 (POU3F4). However, various mutations have been demonstrated in different individuals, which may account for the clinical heterogeneity of DFN3 patients. In fact, this mixed type of hearing impairment is characterized by both conductive hearing impairment resulting from stapes fixation and progressive sensorineural loss of various degrees, and sometimes a profound sensorineural hearing impairment masks the conductive element. Computerized tomography demonstrates abnormal dilatation of the internal acoustic canal, as well as an abnormally wide communication between the internal acoustic canal and the inner ear compartment. As a result, there is increased perilymphatic pressure, which is thought to underlie the observed 'gusher' during the opening of the stapes footplate.

Lalwani et al. (1994) have identified a family with X-linked non-syndromal dominant sensorineural hearing impairment, characterized by incomplete penetrance and variable expressivity in carrier females, and which is linked to the Xp21.2. The auditory impairment in affected males is congenital, bilateral, profound, sensorineural, affecting all frequencies, and without evidence of any radiological abnormality of the temporal bone. Adult carrier females show bilateral, mild-to-moderate high-frequency sensorineural hearing impairment of delayed onset during adulthood. This condition was named DFN4 because it seems different from all other conditions described previously.

The last X-linked condition was described by Del Castillo et al. (1996) who reported a Spanish family affected by a previously undescribed X-linked form of hearing impairment. Hearing impairment was non-syndromal, sensorineural, and progressive. In affected males, the auditory impairment is first detected at school age, affecting mainly the high frequencies. Later it progresses to severe or profound, involving all frequencies. Carrier females show a moderate hearing impairment in the high frequencies, with the onset delayed to the fourth decade of life. The hearing impairment was assumed to be X-linked dominant, with incomplete penetrance and variable expressivity in carrier females.

As with the other types of inheritance, X-linked conditions present with a wide range of possible clinical presentations as well as mutations and genes involved. Even within the same family, clinical heterogeneity can be seen due to variable penetrance and/or environmental factors. The association between sensorineural hearing loss and conductive hearing impairment with malformations of the inner ear should also be remembered. Once again, it is of great importance to collect detailed clinical history and testing in order to contribute to the clinical differentiation of these conditions.

Table 16.1: Non-syndromal X-Linked hearing impairment

Non-Syndromal Hearing Impairment	
Non-Syndromal Hearing Impairment	
Condition: **DFN1**	MIM No:
X-linked syndromal	
Gene Localization: **Xq22**	Gene Identification:
Mutations identified:	
Geographical location of families:	
Ethnic origins of families:	
Detailed origin of families:	
Hearing Impairment	
Penetrance:	
Pathology:	
Type:	
Severity:	
Configuration: [1]	
Unilateral/Bilateral [1]	
Age of onset:	
Progression: [2]	
Interfamilial variability:	
Tinnitus:	
Vestibular function:	
Source References for	
1. Gene localization & identification	
2. Hearing Impairment descriptors	
Contributor & address:	
	Date: 3/4/98
Footnotes: 1. This should include information on its variability. 2. If present define pattern and rate of progression.	

Non-Syndromal Hearing Impairment	
Condition: **DFN2**	MIM No: **304500**
X-linked (dominant?)	
Gene Localization: **Xq22**	Gene Identification: **Unknown**
Mutations identified: **Unknown**	
Geographical location of families: **USA/UK**	
Ethnic origins of families:**Unspecified**	
Detailed origin of families: **Unspecified**	
Hearing Impairment	
Penetrance: **Complete in affected males; incomplete in female carriers**	
Pathology: **Unknown**	
Type: **Cochlear**	
Severity: **Variable: severe/profound in affected males; mild/moderate in female carriers**	
Configuration: [1] **All frequencies in affected males; sloping to high frequencies in carrier females**	
Bilateral	
Age of onset: **Reported as prelingual (congenital?)**	
Progression: [2] **Stable**	
Interfamilial variability: **Unknown**	
Tinnitus: **Unknown**	
Vestibular function: **Unknown**	
Source References for	
1. Gene localization & identification	
• **Tyson et al (1996) Hum Mol Gen, 5, 2055-2060**	
2. Hearing Impairment descriptors	
• **Tyson et al (1996) Hum Mol Gen, 5, 2055-2060**	
Contributor & address:	
Eva Orzan, **Servizio di Audiologia- Università** **di Padova**	Date: **20/4/98**
Footnotes: 1. This should include information on its variability. 2. If present define pattern and rate of progression.	

Non-Syndromal Hearing Impairment	
Condition: **DFN3**	MIM No: **304400**
X-linked	
Gene Localization: **Xq21**	Gene Identification: **POU3F4**
Mutations identified: **L298stop, D215stop, K202stop, L317W, K334E**	
Geographical location of families: **Unspecified**	
Ethnic origins of families: **Caucasoid**	
Detailed origin of families: **Unspecified**	
Hearing Impairment	
Penetrance: **Incomplete in carrier females**	
Pathology: Bony defect (abnormal dilatation of internal acoustic canal and abnormally wide communication between IAC and inner ear compartment) with consequent increased perilymphatic pressure	
Type: **Mixed**	
Severity: **Variable; severe in affected males**	
Configuration: [1] **Variable**	
Bilateral	
Age of onset: **Birth to 10 yrs in affected males; unspecified in affected females**	
Progression: [2] **Progressive**	
Interfamilial variability: **Yes**	
Tinnitus: **Variable manifestation**	
Vestibular function: **Abnormal**	
Source References for	
1. Gene localization & identification	
• **De Kok et al. (1995), Science, 267, 685-688**	
2. Hearing Impairment descriptors	
• **Cremers et al (1985) Arch Otolaryngol 11, 245-254**	
• **Reardon et al. (19919 Genomics 11, 885-894**	
Contributor & address:	
Eva Orzan **Servizio di Audiologia** **Università di Padova**	Date: **20/4/98**
Footnotes: 1. This should include information on its variability. 2. If present define pattern and rate of progression.	

Non-Syndromal Hearing Impairment	
Condition: **DFN4**	MIM No: **300030**
X-linked dominant	
Gene Localization: **Xq21.1**	Gene Identification: **Unknown**
Mutations identified: **Unknown**	
Geographical location of families: **Unspecified (USA?)**	
Ethnic origins of families: **Unspecified**	
Detailed origin of families: **Unspecified**	
Hearing Impairment	
Penetrance: **Incomplete penetrance and variable expressivity in carrier females**	
Pathology: **Unknown**	
Type: **Cochlear**	
Severity: **Profound in affected males; mild/moderate in affected women**	
Configuration: [1] **All frequencies; high frequencies sloping in carrier females**	
Bilateral	
Age of onset: **Uncertain**	
Progression: [2] **Unspecified**	
Interfamilial variability: **Unspecified**	
Tinnitus: **Unspecified**	
Vestibular function: **Unspecified**	
Source References for	
1. Gene localization & identification	
• **Lalwani et al. (1994) Am J Hum Genet 55, 685-694**	
2. Hearing Impairment descriptors	
• **Lalwani et al. (1994) Am J Hum Genet 55, 685-694**	
Contributor & address:	
Eva Orzan, **Servizio di Audiologia** **Università di Padova**	Date: **20/4/98**
Footnotes: 1. This should include information on its variability. 2. If present define pattern and rate of progression.	

Non-Syndromal Hearing Impairment	
Condition: **DFN6**	MIM No: **300066**
X-linked dominant	
Gene Localization: **Xp22**	Gene Identification: **Unknown**
Mutations identified: **Unknown**	
Geographical location of families: **Spain**	
Ethnic origins of families: **Unspecified**	
Detailed origin of families: **Unspecified**	
Hearing Impairment	
Penetrance: **Complete in affected males, incomplete penetrance in carrier females**	
Pathology: **Unknown**	
Type: **Cochlear**	
Severity: **Severe/profound in affected males; moderate in affected females**	
Configuration: [1] All frequencies with sloping to high frequencies at onset in affected males; high frequencies in affected females	
Bilateral	
Age of onset: **Birth to 10 yrs for affected males, 31 to 50 yrs in affected females**	
Progression: [2] Progressive; severe/profound by adulthood in affected males; unspecified for affected females	
Interfamilial variability: **Unknown**	
Tinnitus: **Absent**	
Vestibular function: **Normal**	
Source References for 1. Gene localization & identification • **Del Castillo et al. (1996) Hum Mol Genet, 5, 1383-1387** 2. Hearing Impairment descriptors • **Del Castillo et al. (1996) Hum Mol Genet, 5, 1383-1387**	
Contributor & address: **Eva Orzan, Servizio di Audiologia Università di Padova**	Date: **20/4/98**
Footnotes: 1. This should include information on its variability. 2. If present define pattern and rate of progression.	

References

Cremers CWRJ, Huygen PLM (1983) Clinical features of female heterozygotes in the X-linked mixed deafness syndrome (with perilymphatic gusher during stapes surgery). Int J Pediat Otorhinolaryng 6: 179–185.

Del Castillo I, Villamar M, Sarduy M, Romero L, Herraiz C, Hernandez JH, Rodriguez M, Borras I, Montero A, Bellon J, Tapia MC, Moreno, F (1996) A novel locus for non-syndromic sensorineural deafness (DFN6) maps to chromosome Xp22. Hum Molec Genet 5: 1383–7.

Jin H, May M, Tranebjaerg L, Kendall E, Fontan G, Jackson J, Subramony SH, Arena F, Lubs H, Smith S, Stevenson R, Schwartz C, Vetrie D (1996) A novel X-linked gene, DDP, shows mutations in families with deafness (DFN-1), dystonia, mental deficiency and blindness. Nature Genet 14: 177–80.

Koehler CM, Leuenberger D, Merchant S, Renold A, Junne T, Schatz G (1999) Human deafness dystonia syndrome is a mitochondrial disease. Proc Nat Acad Sci 96: 2141–69.

De Kok YJM, Van der Maarel SM, Bitner-Glindzicz M, Huber I, Monaco AP, Malcolm S, Pembrey ME, Ropers H-H, Cremers FPM (1995) Association between X-linked mixed deafness and mutations in the POU domain gene POU3F4. Science 267: 685–8.

Lalwani AK, Brister JR, Fex J, Grundfast KM, Pikus AT, Ploplis B, San/Agustin T, Skarka H, Wilcox ER (1994) A new nonsyndromic X-linked sensorineural hearing impairment linked to Xp21.2. Am J Hum Genet 55: 685–94.

Mohr J, Mageroy K (1960) Sex-linked deafness of a possibly new type. Acta Genet Statist Med 10: 54–62.

Phelps PD, Reardon W, Pembrey M, Bellman S, Luxon L (1991) X-linked deafness, stapes gushers and a distinctive defect of the inner ear. Neuroradiology 33: 326–30.

Tranebjaerg L, Schwartz C, Eriksen H, Andreasson S, Ponjavic V, Dahl A, Stevenson RE, May M, Arena F, Barker D, Elverland HH, Lubs H (1995) A new X linked recessive deafness syndrome with blindness, dystonia, fractures, and mental deficiency is linked to Xq22. J Med Genet 32: 257–63.

Tranebjaerg L, Van Ghelue M, Nilssen O, Hodes ME, Dlouhy SR, Farlow MR, Hamel B, Arts WFM, Jankovic J, Beach J, Jensen PKA (1997) Jensen syndrome is allelic to Mohr-Tranebjaerg syndrome and both are caused by stop mutations in the DDP gene. (Abstract) Am J Hum Genet 61 (suppl.): A349 only.

Tyson J, Bellman S, Newton V, Simpson P, Malcolm S, Pembrey ME, Bitner-Glindzicz M (1996) Mapping of DFN2 to Xq22. Hum Molec Genet 5: 2055–2060.

Vetrie D, Vorechovsky I, Sideras P, Holland J, Davies A, Flinter F, Hammarstrom L, Kinnon C, Levinsky R, Bobrow M, Smith CIE, Bentley DR (1993) The gene involved in X-linked agammaglobulinaemia is a member of the src family of protein-tyrosine kinases. Nature 361: 226–33.

Chapter 17
Phenotype/genotype correlation of hearing impairment associated with mitochondrial DNA mutations

Howard Jacobs

Introduction

Mitochondrial DNA mutations are associated with both syndromal and non-syndromal forms of hearing impairment, but the relationship between the mitochondrial genotype and clinical phenotype is far from straightforward. A good example (Van den Ouweland et al., 1992; Jean-Francois et al., 1994; and Mariotti et al., 1995) is the well-studied mutation at np 3243 in the gene for tRNA-leu(UUR). This mutation is associated with at least three broadly distinct clinical phenotypes:

- diabetes and/or hearing loss, with no trace of muscle pathology
- ocular myopathy (PEO) with no signs of endocrinopathy or auditory involvement, and
- the full MELAS syndrome, involving a generalized skeletal myopathy, accompanied by a range of CNS defects manifesting as stroke-like episodes and other kinds of seizures, with hearing loss also usually present.

Different individuals in the same family, even with similar proportions and tissue distributions of np 3243 mutant and wild-type mtDNA, can exhibit the full range of different phenotypes associated with the mutation.

In this brief summary I present some of the factors likely to influence the phenotype in mitochondrial disease, as well as some of the pitfalls in genetic analysis thereof. Note that much of our current understanding comes from laboratory studies in highly artificial cell culture systems. In many cases these merely suggest explanations for phenomena in patients.

A full diagnosis and prognosis that can be applied to individual patients is far off, as is any prospect for therapy or even reliable genetic counselling.

Mitochondrial DNA is generally regarded as genetically uniform within an individual, a condition described as homoplasmy. Heteroplasmy, by contrast, is generally regarded as a hallmark of mitochondrial disease, although it is important to note that some disease mutations, notably those at np 1555, 7445 and 7472, which are associated with hearing impairment, are usually homoplasmic or nearly so (El Schahawi et al., 1997; Prezant et al., 1993; Vernham et al., 1994; Fischel Ghodsian et al., 1995; Tiranti et al., 1995). On the other hand, other cases of heteroplasmy need not be pathological, and a debate continues regarding the true extent of low-level heteroplasmy in 'normal' subjects, especially within the tissues of elderly individuals. Documentation of heteroplasmy cannot be taken as proof of pathogenicity for a novel mutation, unless supported by other kinds of evidence.

Mitochondrial mutations associated with hearing impairment fall into two broad classes:

* point mutations in genes whose products contribute to the mitochondrial translation system, including the small subunit (12S) rRNA, plus several tRNAs, notably lysine, serine (UCN) and leucine (UUR), and
* large-scale genomic rearrangements, which can either be heteroplasmic deletions or alternatively, partial duplications.

Point mutations linked to hearing impairment can be either homoplasmic or heteroplasmic but are almost always (maternally) inherited. New mutations are rare, although not unprecedented, but a rather common finding is that the mother and other maternal relatives are clinically unaffected (or only very mildly affected) but, nevertheless, carry the mutation, albeit at a lower level of heteroplasmy. Rapid shifts in heteroplasmy levels between generations are commonly observed and are the result of a kind of genetic bottleneck in the germ-line, which leads to a rather small number of effective founder mtDNA molecules for each oocyte. These complications mean that absence of maternal family history cannot be regarded as an exclusion criterion for mitochondrial hearing impairment. Furthermore, rearrangement mutations are almost always sporadic, and probably constitute the majority. Note that, although deletions are always heteroplasmic, heteroplasmic mutations of all kinds are typically grossly under-represented in blood. Muscle biopsy followed by Southern blot may be the only reliable test for their presence, and this may present ethical difficulties where there are no clinical symptoms that affect muscle.

The question of syndromal versus non-syndromal mitochondrial hearing impairment is a vexed one. Many individuals with a mtDNA mutation exhibit only a hearing impairment, even though others with exactly the same mutation may suffer from a more wide-ranging, multi-system disorder. The case of the np 3243 mutation has already been mentioned, but the np 7472 mutation may be an even clearer example of this (Verhoeven et al., 1999; Ensink et al., 1998) in that most individuals with the mutation, and indeed whole families, are entirely free of neuro-logical defects that characterize the full syndrome of hearing loss, ataxia and myoclonus that has been attributed to the mutation. On the other hand, some features of a syndromal disorder can be easily overlooked, a clear case being that of the np 7445 mutation, which initially was thought to be associated with a purely non-syndromal hearing impairment. Subsequent studies revealed that the mutation is really associated with a syndrome of hearing impairment plus palmoplantar keratoderma (Sevior et al., 1998; plus our unpublished data). Audiologists do not usually examine or even ask about patients' feet, so it is easy to see how this was overlooked.

The phenotypic expression of mitochondrial mutations depends on many factors, although the physical basis of many of them has not yet been fully elucidated. One such set of factors are environmental modifiers, the most clear-cut example being treatment with aminoglycoside antibiotics, which in at least a subset of patients with the np 1555 mutation appears to be an essential cofactor in the development of hearing loss (Prezant et al, 1993).

Mutant gene dosage in heteroplasmic mtDNA disease is also clearly of great importance, although the relationship is rather less clear cut. Typically, below a threshold of 80% to 90% for a given mtDNA mutation, a person may be completely asymptomatic, or at least suffer only a mild hearing impairment. The same phenomenon can be observed in cell culture models in which patient-derived mtDNA is transferred to a control nuclear background at different heteroplasmy levels by cybridization. A549 lung carcinoma cybrids with the np 3243 mutation show a frank respiratory impairment only at mutant dosages of 90% or greater (El Meziane et al., 1998). The exact figure varies between different mtDNA mutations, however. It is probably higher, for example, for those mutations such as np 7472 or 7445 that are usually found in patients as homoplasmic or nearly so. By contrast, much lower levels of heteroplasmy (for example 50%) are clearly pathological in some individuals with the np 3243 mutation, although specific disease features might manifest only where the level of mutant has risen above a higher threshold in some specific cells or tissues. However, there is little experimental evidence in support of this idea, and hence no clear consensus in the field as to the relationship, if any, between tissue distribution of mutant mtDNA and disease phenotype.

Probably a major influence in all cases comes from mtDNA haplotype: the spectrum of other polymorphisms present in the mtDNA of the given family or individual, leaving aside, for the moment, the question of low-level heteroplasmy. In isolation, such polymorphisms are not themselves pathological, but they may influence, either positively or negatively, the clinical expression of *bona fide* disease mutations. A good case in point is the np 7445 mutation, where two different maternal pedigrees have been studied in some detail, both clinically (Vernham et al., 1994; Fischel Ghodsian et al., 1995) and biochemically (Reid et al., 1997; Guan et al., 1998). The two families differ at 10 other nucleotide positions, some of them unique polymorphisms not reported elsewhere. These represent a plausible explanation for the fact that the two families differ both in clinical severity and biochemical phenotype. Most members of one family have a moderate or severe hearing impairment, whereas the other family typically shows only mild hearing impairment, with many unaffected individuals. A very clear example of a dramatic effect of mitochondrial haplotype was revealed by the discovery of the np 12300 suppressor mutation (El Meziane et al., 1998). Low-level heteroplasmy for this tRNA anticodon mutation effectively compensates for the np 3243 mutation in cell culture by replacing the missing tRNA function with a novel one. Although this is a dramatic example not so far actually seen in a patient, it does create a paradigm for understanding the potentially major modifying effects of second-site mutations that may be carried or may arise spontaneously at a low level in patients.

Nuclear genetic background can also have drastic effects on mtDNA disease phenotypes. The most extreme cases are mtDNA aberrations driven by the nuclear genotype. For example, the presence of pathological, multiple mtDNA deletions, generated *de novo* in each generation, is inherited as an autosomal trait, with several different loci involved (Zeviani et al., 1997). A more subtle but still clear influence of nuclear background is evident from cell culture studies, which indicate that the direction of segregation (towards or away from mutant, for a given mtDNA mutation) in heteroplasmic cybrids depends systematically upon the nuclear background of the recipient cell (Dunbar et al., 1995). Furthermore, we found recently that rapid mitotic segregation could occur in heteroplasmic cybrid cells, apparently in response to a nuclear genetic change (Lehtinen et al., 1999). A need for co-operation between nuclear and mitochondrial DNA in the expression of an overt pathological phenotype has also been inferred for families with the np 1555 mutations that contain multiple members with hearing impairment but that have not been treated with aminoglycosides (El Schahawi et al., 1997; Matthijs et al., 1996; Estivill et al., 1998).

Cybrid nuclear background also influences the fate of rearranged mtDNA molecules. For example, in the A549 lung carcinoma background a partial mtDNA duplication is systematically lost by recombination, whereas in the 143B osteosarcoma cell background it is retained (Holt et al., 1997). Such effects in patients can have potentially profound effects on the tissue distribution and hence phenotypic expression of mtDNA rearrangement mutations.

Our own work in np 7472 cybrid cells has revealed an additional level of complexity in that the expression of the biochemical phenotype depends on mtDNA copy number (Toompuu et al, in preparation). An overt phenotype appears only in cell clones with a decreased copy number *and* the mutation. This begs the question of how the mtDNA copy number is regulated in any cell, which remains completely unknown, but once again offers a paradigm for understanding aspects of phenotypic variability between different tissues or different individuals, with a possible contribution from epigenetic as well as nuclear and mitochondrially inherited traits.

It is a truism of medical biology that 'more research is needed' in order to enable clinicians to make useful judgements about diagnosis and treatment. Mitochondrial disease genetics, particularly concerning mutations, which affect the auditory system, is a very clear example. In fact, we remain completely ignorant of the primary mechanism by which defects in mitochondrial translation cause hearing loss. Ten competing hypotheses are still viable. We require a model system that can enable us to investigate them at the whole organism level, which for mitochondrial mutations is a far from trivial undertaking.

Table 17.1: Non-syndromal hearing impairment forms

Non-Syndromal Hearing Impairment	
Condition: **Maternally-inherited,non aminoglycoside-induced**	MIM No:590080 **(allelic variant 002)**
Mitochondrial	
Gene Location: **Mt 7445**	Gene Identification: **serine-tRNA**
Mutations identified: **T7445C**	
Geographical location of families: **Scotland, New Zealand**	
Ethnic origins of families: **Caucasoid**	
Detailed origin of families: **West Scotland (Glasgow)**	
Hearing Impairment	
Penetrance: **Incomplete** in the Scottish pedigree, **Complete** in the New Zealand one	
Pathology: **Unknown**	
Type: **Cochlear**	
Severity: **Mild to severe**	
Configuration: [1] **High frequencies**	
Bilateral	
Age of onset: [2] **11 to 30 years**	
Progression: [3] **Progressive**	
Interfamilial variability: **Unknown**	
Tinnitus: **Unknown**	
Vestibular function: **Unknown**	
Source References for	

1. Gene location & identification

- *Reid FM, Vernham GA, Jacobs HT. Hum Molec Genet 3, 1435-6, 1994.*

2. Hearing loss descriptors

- *Reid FM, Vernham GA, Jacobs HT. Hum Mutation 3, 243-7, 1994;*
- *Reardon W, Harding AE. Review: J Audio Med 4, 40-51, 1995;*
- *Fischel-Ghodsian N. Bull Nat Inst on Deafness and Other Communication Disorders 2, 1996;*
- *Fischel-Ghodsian N et al. Am J Otolaryngol 16, 1995.*

Contributor & address:

G. Lina-Granade, Department of   **Date:** 30/3/1998
ORL, Hopital E. Herriot, Lyon, France.

Non-Syndromal Hearing Impairment	
Condition: **Maternally-inherited or sporadic, aminoglycoside-induced or not**	MIM No: **580000 and 561000 +/– 221745**
Mitochondrial +/– Autosomal Recessive	
Gene Location: **Mt 1555**	Gene Identification: **12S ribosomal RNA**
Mutations identified: **A1555G**	
Geographical location of families: **Israel, Japan, China, Zaire, Spain, Cuba**	
Ethnic origins of families: **Caucasoid, Mongoloid, Negroid**	
Detailed origin of families: **Arabic from Israel, Shanghai (China), Mayombe (South-West Zaire)**	
Hearing Impairment Penetrance: **Incomplete**	
Pathology: **Unknown**	
Type: **Cochlear**	
Severity: **Mild to profound**	
Configuration: [1] **High frequencies (when specified)**	
Unilateral/bilateral: **Bilateral**	
Age of onset: [2] **Variable (congenital, 1st decade, 2nd to 4th decade)**	
Progression: [3] **Progressive when non-congenital**	
Interfamilial variability: **Yes (highly heterogeneous)**	
Tinnitus: **Variable manifestation or unknown**	
Vestibular function: **Clinically normal**	
Source References for **1. Gene location & identification:** • *Prezant TR et al. Nature Genet 4, 289-93, 1993.* • *Hutchin T et al. Nucleic Acid Research 21, 4174-9, 1993.* • *Fischel-Ghodsian N et al. Am J Otolaryngol 14, 399-403, 1993.* **1. Hearing loss descriptors:** • *Jaber L et al. J Med Genet 29, 86-90, 1992.* • *El-Schahawi M et al. Neurology 45, Suppl 4, Abstract 1006P, 1995.* • *Tamagawa Y et al. Acta Otolaryngol 116, 796-8, 1996.* • *Matthijs G et al. Eur J Hum Genet 4, 46-51, 1996.*	

(contd)

- *Tsuiki et al. Ann Otol Rhinol Laryngol 106, 643-8, 1997.*
- *Sarduy M et al. Stephens D, Read A, Martini A, eds. Developments in Genetic Hearing Impairment I. London: Whurr (1999).*
- *Reardon W, Harding AE. J Audiol Med 4, 40-51, 1995.*
- *Fischel-Ghodsian N. Bulletin of the National Institute on Deafness and Other Communication Disorders 2, 1996.*

Contributor & address:	
G. Lina-Granade, Department of ORL, Hopital E. Herriot, Lyon, France.	Date: 30/3/98

References

Dunbar DR, Moonie PA, Young H, Jacobs HT, Holt IJ (1995) Different cellular backgrounds confer a marked advantage to either mutant or wild-type mitochondrial genomes. Proceedings of the National Academy Science USA 92, 6562–6.

El Meziane A, Lehtinen S, Hance N, Nijtmans LGJ, Dunbar D, Holt IJ, Jacobs HT (1998) A tRNA suppressor mutation in human mitochondria. Nature Genetics 18: 350–3.

El Schahawi M, deMunain AL, Sarrazin AM, Shanske AL, Basirico M, Shanske S, DiMauro S (1997) Two large Spanish pedigrees with nonsyndromic sensorineural deafness and the mtDNA mutation at nt 1555 in the 12S rRNA gene. Evidence of Heteroplasmy 48, 453–6.

Ensink RJH, Verhoeven K, Marres HAM, Huygen PLM, Padberg GW, Ter Laak H, Van Camp G, Willems PJ, Cremers CWRJ. (1998) Early-onset sensorineural hearing loss and late-onset neurologic complaints caused by a mitochondrial mutation at position 74-72. Archives of Otolaryngology-Head and Neck Surgery 124: 886–91.

Estivill X, Govea N, Barcelo A, Percllo E, Badenas C, Romero E, Moral L, Scozzari R, Durbano L, Zeviani M, Torroni A (1998) Familial progressive sensorineural deafness is mainly due to the mtDNA A1555G mutation and is enhanced by treatment with aminoglycosides. American Journal of Human Genetics 62: 27–35.

Fischel Ghodsian N, Prezant TR, Fourier P, Stewart IA, Maw M (1995) Mitochondrial mutation associated with nonsyndromic deafness. American Journal of Otolaryngology 16: 403–8.

Guan MX, Enriquez JA, Fischel Ghodsian N, Puranam RS, Lin CP, Maw MA, Attardi G (1998) The deafness-associated mitochondrial DNA mutation at position 7445, which affects tRNA(Ser(UCN)) precursor processing, has long-range effects on NADH dehydrogenase subunit ND6 gene expression. Molecular and Cellular Biology 18: 5868–79.

Holt IJ, Dunbar DR, Jacobs HT (1997) Behaviour of a population of partially duplicated mitochondrial DNA molecules in cell culture: segregation, maintenance and recombination dependent upon nuclear background. Human and Molecular Genetics 6: 1251–60.

Jean-Francois MJB, Lertrit P, Berkovic SF, Crimmins D, Morris J, Marzuki S, Byrne E (1994) Heterogeneity in the phenotypic-expression of the mutation in the mitochondrial tRNA(leu(UUR)) gene generally associated with the MELAS subset of mitochondrial encephalomyopathies. Australian New Zealand Journal of Medicine 24, 188–93.

Lehtinen SK, Hance N, El Meziane A, Juhola MK, Juhola KMI, Karhu R, Spelbrink JN, Holt IJ and Jacobs HT (1999) Genotypic stability, segregation and selection in heteroplasmic human cell-lines containing np 3243 mutant mtDNA. Genetics (submitted)

Mariotti C, Savarese N, Suomalainen A, Rimoldi M, Comi G, Prelle A, Antozzi C, Servidei S, Jarre L, Di Donato S, Zeviani M (1995) Genotype to phenotype correlations in mitochondrial encephalomyopathies associated with the A3243G mutation of mitochondrial DNA. Journal of Neurology 242: 304–12.

Matthijs G, Claes S, LongoMbenza B, Cassiman JJ (1996) Non-syndromic deafness associated with a mutation and a polymorphism in the mitochondrial 12S ribosomal RNA gene in a large Zairean pedigree. European Journal of Human Genetics 4: 46–51.

Prezant TR, Agapian JV, Bohlman MC, Bu X, Oztas S, Qiu WQ, Arnos KS, Cortopassi GA, Jaber L,

Rotter JI, Shohat M, Fischel-Ghodsian N (1993) Mitochondrial ribosomal RNA mutation associated with both antibiotic-induced and non-syndromic deafness. Nature Genetics 4: 289–94.

Reid FM, Rovio A, Holt IJ, Jacobs HT (1997) Molecular phenotype of a human lymphoblastoid cell-line homoplasmic for the np 7445 deafness-associated mitochondrial mutation. Human Molecular Genetics 6: 443–9.

Sevior KB, Hatamochi A, Stewart IA, Bykhovskaya Y, AllenPowell DR, Fischel Ghodsian N, Maw MA (1998) Mitochondrial A7445G mutation in two pedigrees with palmoplantar keratoderma and deafness. American Journal of Medical Genetics 75: 179–85.

Tiranti V, Chariot P, Carella F, Toscano A, Soliveri P, Girlanda P, Carrara F, Fratta GM, Reid FM, Mariotti C, Zeviani M (1995) Maternally inherited hearing loss, ataxia and myoclonus associated with a novel point mutation in mitochondrial tRNA(SER(UCN)) gene. Human Molecular Genetics 4: 1421–7.

Van den Ouweland JMW, Lemkes HHPG, Ruitenbeek W, Sandkjujl LA, DeVijlder MF, Struyvenberg PAA, Van de Kamp JJP, Maassen JA (1992) Mutation in mitochondrial transfer RNA (Leu(UUR)) gene in a large pedigree with maternally transmitted type II diabetes mellitus and deafness. Nature Genetics 1: 368–71.

Verhoeven K, Ensink RJH, Tiranti V, Huygen PLM, Johnson DF, Schatteman I, VanLaer L, Verstreken M, VandeHeyning P, Fischel Ghodsian N, Zeviani M, Cremers CWRJ, Willems PJ, VanCamp G (1999) Hearing impairment and neurological dysfunction associated with a mutation in the mitochondrial tRNA(Ser(UCN)) gene. European Journal of Human Genetics 7: 45–51.

Vernham GA, Reid FM, Rundle PA, Jacobs HT (1994) Bilateral sensorineural hearing loss in members of a maternal lineage with a mitochondrial point mutation. Clinical Otolaryngology 19: 314–19.

Zeviani M, Petruzzella V, Carrozzo R (1997) Disorders of nuclear-mitochondrial intergenomic signalling. Journal of Bioenergetics and Biomembranes 29: 121–30.

Part IV
Relevant Websites

Chapter 18
The hereditary hearing loss homepage

(URL:http://www.via.ac.be/dnalab/hhh/)

GUY VAN CAMP, RICHARD JH SMITH

In 1994–5, as the number of reported loci for non-syndromal hearing impairment quickly increased, it became apparent that a rapid means of exchange of information was needed to avoid confusion in nomenclature. In November 1995, a list of known loci with their correct nomenclature was placed on the Internet under the name 'hereditary hearing loss homepage'. Although initially a simple table containing locus names, cytogenetic localizations, screening markers and references, the resource has grown to include various other types of information, such as information on cloned genes, links to other databases, and syndromal hearing impairment.

Although both syndromal and non-syndromal hearing impairment are covered in the homepage, the main focus is non-syndromal hearing impairment. This paper provides brief descriptions of known genes for non-syndromal hearing impairment, and presents parts of tables found in the homepage (Tables 18.1 to 18.4). For more information, such as screening markers, references, information on syndromal hearing impairment and links to OMIM and PubMed, please consult the homepage online.

The hereditary hearing loss homepage can be reached at the following URL address:

http://www.uia.ac.be/dnalab/hhh/

COCH (DFNA9) – The *COCH* gene was isolated from a human foetal cochlear cDNA library and is expressed at high levels in the cochlear and vestibular system. *In situ* hybridization in the chicken cochlear and vestibular organs shows localization of Coch mRNA in the support structures and neural channels within these labyrinths (Robertson et

Table 18.1: Gene localizations for autosomal dominant non-syndromic hearing impairment

Locus Name	Location	Gene
DFNA1	5q31	HDIA1
DFNA2	1p34	GJB3, KCNQ4
DFNA3	13q12	GJB2, GJB6
DFNA4	19q13	Unknown
DFNA5	7p15	DFNA5
DFNA6	4p16.3	Unknown
DFNA7	1q21-q23	Unknown
DFNA8	11q22-24	TECTA
DFNA9	14q12-q13	COCH
DFNA10	6q22-q23	Unknown
DFNA11	11q12.3-q21	MYO7A
DFNA12	11q22-q24	TECTA
DFNA13	6p21	COL11A2
DFNA14	4p16	Unknown
DFNA15	5q31	POU4F3
DFNA16	2q24	Unknown
DFNA17	22q	Unknown
DFNA18	3q22	Unknown
DFNA19	10 (pericentr.)	Unknown
DFNA20	17q25	Unknown
DFNA21	Reserved	
DFNA22	Reserved	
DFNA23	14q	Unknown
DFNA24	4q	Unknown
DFNA25	12q21-24	Unknown
DFNA26	17q25	Unknown
DFNA27	4q12	Unknown
DFNA28	8q22	Unknown
DFNA29	Reserved	
DFNA30	15q26	Unknown
DFNA31	Reserved	

al., 1998). These areas correspond to human inner ear structures in which acidophilic deposits are seen in persons with DFNA9 hearing impairment (Khetarpal et al., 1991; Khetarpal, 1993). The region of *COCH* harbouring three missense mutations in three American *DFNA9* families shows homology to a domain of unknown function in factor C in the horseshoe crab, *Limulus*, which upon binding with lipopolysac-charides initiates a coagulation cascade (Robertson et al., 1998). Another mutation in the factor C domain (P51S) seems to be particu-larly frequent in Belgium and the Netherlands (de Kok et al, 1999;

Table 18.2: Gene localizations for autosomal recessive non-syndromic hearing impairment

Locus Name	Location	Gene
DFNB1	13q12	*GJB2*
DFNB2	11q13.5	*MYO7A*
DFNB3	17p11.2	*MYO15*
DFNB4	7q31	*PDS*
DFNB5	14q12	Unknown
DFNB6	3p14-p21	Unknown
DFNB7	9q13-q21	Unknown
DFNB8	21q22	Unknown
DFNB9	2p22-p23	*OTOF*
DFNB10	21q22.3	*TMPRSS3*
DFNB11	9q13-q21	Unknown
DFNB12	10q21-q22	Unknown
DFNB13	7q34-36	Unknown
DFNB14	7q31	Unknown
DFNB15	3q21-25 and 19p13	Unknown
DFNB16	15q21-q22	Unknown
DFNB17	7q31	Unknown
DFNB18	11p14-15.1	Unknown
DFNB19	18p11	Unknown
DFNB20	11q25-qter	Unknown
DFNB21	11q	*TECTA*
DFNB22	Reserved	
DFNB23	10p11.2-q21	Unknown
DFNB24	11q23	Unknown
DFNB25	4p15.3-q12	Unknown
DFNB26	4q2 and 1q22-23	Unknown
DFNB27	Reserved	
DFNB28	22q13	Unknown

Fransen et al, 1999). *DFNA9* is currently the only autosomal dominant non-syndromal hearing impairment locus reported to involve vestibular symptoms, and Fransen et al, (1999) have reported additional symptoms of Menière's disease (vertigo, tinnitus, aural fullness) in more than 25% of patients with a *COCH* mutation.

DFNA5 – The *DFNA5* gene is expressed in the cochlea and several other tissues. It shows no significant homology to any other known gene, and no clues as to its function could be found despite extensive computational analysis. *DFNA5* is likely identical to the *ICERE1* gene, a gene that is up-regulated in oestrogen receptor-negative breast carcinomas

Table 18.3: Gene localizations for X-linked non-syndromic hearing

Locus Name	Location	Gene
DFN1	Xq22	DDP
DFN2	Xq22	Unknown
DFN3	Xq21.1	POU3F4
DFN4	Xp21.2	Unknown
DFN5	Symbol withdrawn	
DFN6	Xp22	Unknown
DFN7	Symbol withdrawn	
DFN8	Reserved	

*Restudy of the original *DFN1* family showed that the deafness is part of a progressive X-linked recessive syndrome, which includes visual disability, dystonia, fractures and mental deficiency. Therefore, *DFN1* is a syndromic form of deafness and does not actually belong in the list of nonsyndromic forms of deafness.

Table 18.4: Mitochondrial mutations leading to non-syndromic hearing impairment

Gene	Mutation
12SrRNA	1555A(G)
tRNA-Ser(UCN)	7445A(G)

(Thompson et al, 1998). Definitive proof of the involvement of the *ICERE1* gene in breast cancer pathogenesis is lacking, and it is possible that up-regulation of *ICERE1* in oestrogen receptor-negative breast carcinomas is a side effect rather than a causative factor of tumour formation (Van Laer et al., 1998). A complex mutation in intron 7, involving a deletion of 1189 bp, a small insertion derived from intron 8, and a GCCCA-stretch from unknown origin, was found in a single extended Dutch family (Van Laer et al., 1998). On the mRNA level, exon 8 is skipped, leading to a frame shift and a predicted premature truncation of the protein.

DIAPH1 (DFNA1) – The human *DFNA1* protein product DIAPH1, mouse p140mDia, and *Drosophila diaphanous* are homologues of *Saccharomyces cerevisiae* protein Bni1p. These proteins are highly conserved and belong to the formin family. All formins share N-terminal Rho-binding domains, central polyproline stretches, and C-terminal formin-homology domains. Rho regulates actin polymerization, which may be particularly important for hair cells. Other functions involve cytokinesis and establishment of cell polarity. *DIAPH1* is expressed in multiple tissues, including brain, heart, placenta, lung, kidney, pancreas, liver and skeletal muscle. Lynch et al. (1997) found a splice site mutation leading to a frameshift in the *DIAPH1* mRNA in a large Costa Rican kindred linked to *DFNA1*.

Gap junction proteins – GJB2 (*DFNB1* and *DFNA3*), GJB3 (*DFNA2*), and GJB6 (*DFNA3*). Gap junctions are plasma membrane channels formed by six sub-unit proteins called connexins. The formation of intercellular channels is possible through interaction with connexins in the plasma membrane of adjacent cells. Gap junctions are found in many cell types and facilitate the exchange of molecules up to 1 kDa between cells.

GJB2 – The gap junction protein, beta-2 (GJB2) is also called (and probably better known as) Connexin 26 (Cx26). Cx26 is widely expressed in many tissues. Immunohistochemical experiments have shown Cx26 expression in the stria vascularis, basement membrane, limbus and the spiral prominence of the cochlea. At least 21 different disease-causing mutations of Cx26 have been identified that result in autosomal recessive non-syndromal hearing impairment. The most common mutation, 35delG (also called 30delG), occurs in a stretch of 6 G residues at positions 30–35 of the Cx26 DNA sequence. This mutation is found in over two-thirds of persons with *DFNB1* and has been reported in many populations of different ethnicity (Carrasquillo et al., 1997; Denoyelle et al., 1997; Estivill et al., 1998a; Green ct al., 1999; Kelley et al., 1998; Zelante et al., 1997). Although Cx26 mutations are a frequent cause of hearing impairment in the Japanese population, the 35delG mutation is not found (S Usami, personal communication). Kelsell et al. (1997) found a Cx26 missense mutation, M34T, in one autosomal dominant family linked to chromosome 13 (*DFNA3*), and electrophysiological measurements support their hypothesis that it causes hearing loss by a dominant negative effect (White et al., 1998). However, this mutation also has been found in numerous individuals with normal hearing (Scott et al., 1997; Kelley et al., 1998) suggesting that it could represent a rare polymorphism. Another missense mutation, W44C, causes autosomal dominant hearing impairment in two French *DFNA3* families (Denoyelle et al., 1998).

GJB3 – Wenzel et al. (1998) isolated a new gap junction protein (beta-3, GJB3, or connexin 31) that Heller et al. (1998) also identified in an auditory epithelium-specific cDNA library. Subsequently, mutations in this gene were found in families with an autosomal dominant skin disorder called erythrokeratodermia variabilis (Richard et al., 1998), and in two small Chinese families with autosomal dominant non-syndromic hearing impairment (Xia et al., 1998). The mutations in the latter families included a nonsense mutation and a missense mutation that changed a highly conserved residue. These mutations were also present in normally hearing family members implying, at a minimum, reduced penetrance.

GJB6 – In 1999, Grifa et al. cloned the human homologue of mouse gap junction protein beta-6 (Gjb6), a gene tightly linked to Gjb2. Because a number of families linked to the *DFNA3* locus were negative for GJB2 mutations, they hypothesized that mutations might be found in GJB6 and completed a mutation screen on 198 deaf people. One missense mutation was discovered, changing an evolutionarily conserved residue in three deaf people from a single family. Electrophysiological measurements on *Xenopus* oocytes expressing the mutant connexin indicated that the mutation has a dominant negative effect on wild-type channels.

KCNQ4 (*DFNA2*) – A novel potassium channel (KCNQ4), was described recently by Kubisch et al. (1999). KCNQ4 encodes a protein containing six transmembrane domains, a highly conserved P-loop lining the channel pore, and two cytoplasmic domains; four KCNQ4 subunits aggregate to form a functional channel. In a single French family with autosomal dominant non-syndromal hearing impairment, a missense mutation (G285S) was discovered in the highly conserved P-loop of KCNQ4. Oocytes expressing the mutant KCNQ4 protein indicate that this mutation impairs channel function by a dominant-negative effect. KCNQ4 expression has been detected in heart, brain and skeletal muscle by northern blot, and in mouse cochlear and vestibular cells by RT-PCR. *In situ* hybridization revealed that the KCNQ4 message was present only in the outer hair cells of the organ of Corti, suggesting that it might play a role in the recycling of potassium ions in the endolymph after hair-cell stimulation. Coucke et al. (1999) reported KCNQ4 mutations in 4 *DFNA2* families. Two of them are missense mutations in the P-loop domain, one is a missense mutation in the sixth transmembrane domain, and one is a 13-bp deletion expected to lead to a small protein that is truncated before the first transmembrane domain. No KCNQ4 mutation could be found in the original Indonesian *DFNA2* family (Coucke et al, 1999).

Mitochondrial mutations – The 1555AG mutation in the 12S rRNA gene has been found in several families with maternally inherited, non-syndromal hearing impairment, and in people and families with amino-glycoside-induced ototoxic hearing impairment (Prezant et al., 1993; Usami et al., 1997; Estivill et al., 1998b). The mutation makes individuals susceptible to hearing impairment after treatment with aminoglycosides at concentrations that normally do not affect hearing. Even without exposure to aminoglycosides, some mutation carriers develop hearing impairment. The 7445AG mutation was found in a Scottish family and a New Zealand family with maternally inherited, sensorineural hearing impairment (Reid et al., 1994; Fischel-Ghodsian et al., 1995). Clinical re-evaluation of the pedigrees revealed palmoplantar keratoderma in most patients. In addition, the 7445AG mutation was found in a Japanese family with maternally inherited palmoplantar keratoderma and progressive sensorineural hearing impairment (Sevior et al., 1998).

OTOF (*DFNB9*) – The *OTOF* gene is homologous to the *C. Elegans FER-1* gene (Yasunaga et al., 1999), and is predicted to be a cytosolic protein that anchors to the cell membrane through its C-terminal domain. It also contains three C2-domains that interact with phospholipids. Yasunaga et al. hypothesize that otoferlin is involved in trafficking of membrane vesicles, possibly synaptic vesicles. *In situ* hybridization experiments show that OTOF is expressed mainly in inner hair cells and vestibular type I sensory hair cells. A nonsense mutation (Y730X) has been detected in four Lebanese consanguinous families with autosomal recessive non-syndromal severe-to-profound prelingual deafness.

PDS (*DFNB4*, Pendred syndrome) – The *PDS* gene is part of a highly conserved gene family that encodes hydrophobic proteins with the sulphate transporter signature. The predicted amino acid sequence of the PDS gene product (called pendrin) contains 11 transmembrane proteins. Scott et al. (1999) demonstrated that pendrin functions as a transporter of chloride and iodide but not sulphate. Twenty-six different mutations in the *PDS* gene have been reported to cause Pendred syndrome (Everett et al., 1997; Van Hauwe et al., 1998). Four mutations (L236P, E384G, T416P and 1001+1G-to-A) are seen most frequently and together account for 67% of the Pendred disease alleles in patients with a confirmed diagnosis of Pendred syndrome (Coyle et al., 1998; Van Hauwe et al., 1998). Two unique mutations in the *PDS* gene have been reported in a single consanguineous family with autosomal recessive non-syndromal hearing impairment (*DFNB4*), implicating *PDS* in both syndromal and non-syndromal hearing impairment (Li et al., 1998). Affected individuals in the *DFNB4* family had dilated vestibular aqueducts (DVA) and *PDS* mutations have also been found in other people with DVA syndrome (Usami et al, 1999).

POU Genes – *POU3F4* (*DFN3*) and *POU4F3* (*DFNA15*). *POU* genes share a POU-specific domain and a POU homeodomain, both of which are required for high-affinity binding to DNA target sites. The POU region consists of a highly conserved homeodomain of 60 amino acids and a POU-specific domain of 76-78 amino acids. Genes in this family serve as critical developmental regulators for the determination of cellular phenotypes (Ingraham et al., 1990; Rosenfeld, 1991).

POU3F4 – *POU3F4* (class 3, transcription factor 4) was the first autosomal hearing impairment gene to be identified (de Kok et al., 1995). This gene is mutated or deleted in families with X-linked congenital mixed conductive and sensorineural hearing impairment (*DFN 3*). Affected individuals also have stapes fixation and an abnormal communication between the cerebrospinal fluid and perilymph, which may cause leakage during otological surgery (perilymphatic gusher).

POU4F3 – *POU4F3* is another member of the family of POU domain transcription factors (class 4, transcription factor 3). In 'knock-out' mice, targeted mutagenesis of both *Pou4f3* alleles leads to profound hearing impairment and vestibular dysfunction (Erkman et al., 1996). In humans, progressive hearing impairment has been reported in an Israeli family segregating for an 8-base pair deletion in *POU4F3* that forms a mutant truncated protein (*DFNA 15* – Vahava et al. 1998).

TECTA (*DFNA8, DFNA12, DFNB21*) – *TECTA* encodes an extracellular matrix protein (alpha tectorin) that is the main non-collagenous component of the tectorial membrane of the inner ear. Alpha tectorin contains three polypeptide domains: a module containing a region homologous to the G1 domain of entactin, a module similar to zonadhesin (an outer coat sperm protein), and a zona pellucida domain (Verhoeven et al., 1998). The latter were found first in proteins from the zona pellucida (the region surrounding the unfertilized egg). Verhoeven et al. (1998) reported three different missense mutations in two different families with autosomal dominant non-syndromal hearing impairment. In an Austrian *DFNA8* family, a Y1870C mutation was found; in a Belgian *DFNA12* family, L1820F and G1824D mutations were detected. In both families, the hearing impairment is congenital and non-progressive and the mutations lie in the zona pellucida domain. A mutation in the zonadhesin-like domain was reported by Alloisio et al. (1999) in a French family with progressive hearing impairment starting in the high frequencies. Mustapha et al. (1998) described a Lebanese family in which nine individuals had a pre-lingual severe-to-profound non-syndromal hearing impairment. The family showed linkage to chromosome 11q23-25, the region where alpha-tectorin is located. Mutation analysis revealed a splice site mutation leading to a truncated protein. These results indicate that mutations in alpha-tectorin can result in both dominant and recessive forms of hearing impairment.

Unconventional Myosins – *MYO7A* (*DFNB2, DFNA11, USH1B*) and *MYO15* (*DFNB3*). Myosins are divided into subclasses on the basis of comparisons of motor domains and tails. Conventional myosins are class II; the other 14 classes (I, III-XV) are unconventional myosins. Unconventional myosins, such as myosin VIIA, share structurally conserved heads which move along actin filaments using actin-activated ATPase activity, and have divergent tails presumably to move different macromolecular structures relative to actin filaments.

MYO15 – A genetic distance tree constructed with a portion of the motor domains of 40 myosins suggests that MYO15 is sufficiently divergent to constitute a new class of myosins designated myosin XV (Probst et al., 1998). Its coding sequence includes more than 50 exons spanning 36 kilobases. An amino acid substitution at a highly conserved position within the motor domain in the *shaker-2* mouse, the homologue of *DFNB3*, results in hair cells with very short stereocilia and a long actin-containing bundle that protrudes from the basal end (Probst et al., 1998). This finding suggests that MYO15 is necessary for actin organization in hair cells. Two missense mutations (I892P, N890Y) and one nonsense mutation (K1300X) have been found in three *DFNB3* families (Wang et al., 1998).

MYO7A – In the ear, myosin VIIA is present in both inner and outer hair cells, although expression is greater in the former. In the eye, it is localized to microvilli projections in retinal pigmentary epithelial cells and photoreceptor cells (Hasson et al., 1995). Mutations in myosin VIIA have been identified in Usher syndrome type 1b, a recessively inherited disease characterized by congenital deafness, vestibular dysfunction and retinitis pigmentosa (Weil et al., 1995). Myosin VIIA mutations in nonsyndromal hearing impairment (*DFNB2*) were found by Liu et al. (1997a) and by Weil et al. (1997). Recessive mutations in the mouse homologue give rise to the *shaker-1* phenotype, which is characterized by hyperactivity, head-tossing and circling behaviour due to vestibular and cochlear dysfunction (Gibson et al., 1995). A mutation in myosin VIIA has also been found in a Japanese family with autosomal dominant non-syndromal progressive hearing impairment (*DFNA11*, Liu et al., 1997b).

Acknowledgements

This work was supported in part by grants from the Flemish fund for Scientific Research (FWO) and the University of Antwerp to GVC, and grants RO1-DC02842 and RO1-DC03544 (RJHS).

References

Alloisio N, Morle L, Bozon M, Godet J, Verhoeven K, Van Camp G, Plauchu H, Muller P, Collet L, Lina-Granade G (1999) Mutation in the zonadhesin-like domain of a-tectorin associated with autosomal dominant non-syndromic hearing loss. European Journal of Human Genetics 7: 45–51.

Carrasquillo MM, Zlotogora J, Barges S, Chakravarti A (1997) Two different connexin 26 mutations in an inbred kindred segregating non-syndromic recessive deafness: implications for genetic studies in isolated populations. Human Molecular Genetics 6: 2163–72.

Coucke PJ, Van HP, Kelley PM, Kunst H, Schatteman I, Van VD, Meyers J, Ensink RJ, Verstreken M, Declau F, Marres H, Kastury K, Bhasin S, McGuirt WT, Smith RJ, Cremers CW, Van de Heyning PH, Willems PJ, Smith SD, Van Camp G (1999) Mutations in the KCNQ4 gene are responsible for autosomal dominant deafness in four DFNA2 families. Hum Mol Genet 8: 1321–8.

Coyle B, Reardon W, Herbrick JA, Tsui LC, Gausden E, Lee J, Coffey, R., Grueters, A., Grossman, Phelps, P.D., Luxon, L., Kendall-Taylor, P., Scherer, S.W., and Trembath, R.C. (1998) Molecular analysis of the PDS gene in Pendred syndrome. Human Molecular Genetics 7: 1105–12.

De Kok YJ, Bom SJ, Brunt TM, Kemperman MH, Van BE, Van DV, Robertson NG, Morton CC, Huygen PL, Verhagen WI, Brunner HG, Cremers CW, Cremers FP (1999) A Pro51Ser mutation in the COCH gene is associated with late onset autosomal dominant progressive sensorineural hearing loss with vestibular defects.Human Molecular Genetics 8: 361–6.

De Kok YJ, Van der Maarel SM, Bitner-Glindzicz M, Huber I, Monaco AP, Malcolm S, Pembrey ME, Ropers HH, Cremers FP (1995) Association between X-linked mixed deafness and mutations in the POU domain gene POU3F4. Science 267: 685–8.

Denoyelle F, Lina-Granade G, Plauchu H, Bruzzone R, Chaib H, Levi-Acobas F, Weil D, Petit C (1998) Connexin 26 gene linked to a dominant deafness. Nature 393: 319–20.

Denoyelle F, Weil D, Maw MA, Wilcox SA, Lench NJ, Allen-Powell DR, Osborn AH, Dahl HHM, Middleton A, Houseman MJ, Dodé C, Marlin S, Boulila-ElGaïed A, Grati M, Ayadi H, BenArab S, Bitoun P, Lina-Granade G, Godet J, Mustapha M, Loiselet J, El-Zir E, Aubois A, Joannard A, Levilliers J, Garabédian EN, Mueller RF, Gardner RJM, Petit C (1997) Prelingual deafness: high prevalence of a 30delG mutation in the connexin 26 gene. Human Molecular Genetics 6: 2173–7.

Erkman L, McEvilly RJ, Luo L, Ryan AK, Hooshmand F, O'Connell SM, Keithley EM, Rapaport DH, Ryan AF, Rosenfeld MG (1996) Role of transcription factors Brn-3.1 and Brn-3.2 in auditory and visual system development. Nature 381: 603–6.

Estivill X, Fortina P, Surrey S, Rabionet R, Melchionda S, D'Agruma L, Mansfield E, Rappaport E, Govea N, Mila M, Zelante L, Gasparini P (1998a) Connexin-26 mutations in sporadic and inherited sensorineural deafness. Lancet 351: 394–8.

Estivill X, Govea N, Barcelo E, Badenas C, Romero E, Moral L, Scozzri R, D'Urbano L, Zeviani M, Torroni A (1998b) Familial progressive sensorineural deafness is mainly due to the mtDNA A1555G mutation and is enhanced by treatment with aminoglycosides American Journal of Human Genetics 62: 27–35.

Everett, LA, Glazer B, Beck JC, Idol JR, Buchs A, Heyman M, Adawi F, Hazani E, Nassir E, Baxevanis AD, Sheffield VC, Green ED (1997) Pendred syndrome is caused by mutations in a putative sulphate transporter gene (PDS). Nature Genetics 17: 411–22.

Fischel-Ghodsian N, Prezant TR, Fournier P, Stewart IA, Maw M (1995) Mitochondrial mutation associated with nonsyndromic deafness. American Journal of Otolaryngology 16: 403–8.

Fransen E, Verstreken M, Verhagen WIM, Wuyts FL, Huygen PLM, D'Haese P, Robertson NG, Morton CC, McGuirt WT, Smith RJH, Declau F, Van de Heyning PH, Van Camp G (1999) High prevalence of symptoms of Menière's disease in three families with a mutation in the COCH gene. Human Molecular Genetics 8: 1425–9.

Gibson F, Walsh J, Mburu P, Varela A, Brown KA, Antonio M, Beisel KW, Steel KP, Brown SD (1995) A type VII myosin encoded by the mouse deafness gene shaker-1. Nature 374: 62–4.

Green GE, Scott DA, McDonald JM, Woodworth GG, Sheffield VC, Smith RJ (1999) Carrier rates in the mid-western United States for GJB2 mutations causing inherited deafness. Journal of American Medical Association 281: 2211–6.

Grifa A, Wagner CA, D'Ambrosio L, Melchionda S, Bernardi F, Lopez-Bigas N, Rabionet R, Arbones M, Monica MD, Estivill X, Zelante L, Lang F, Gasparini P (1999) Mutations in GJB6 cause nonsyndromic autosomal dominant deafness at DFNA3 locus. Nature Genetics 23: 16–18.

Hasson T, Heintzelman MB, Santos-Sacchi J, Corey DP, Mooseker MS (1995) Expression in cochlea and retina of myosin VIIa, the gene product defective in Usher syndrome type 1B. Proceedings of the National Academy of the USA 92: 9815–19.

Heller S, Sheane CA, Javed Z, Hudspeth AJ (1998) Molecular markers for cell types of the inner ear and candidate genes for hearing disorders. Proc Natl Acad Sci USA 95: 11400–5.

Ingraham HA, Albert VR, Chen RP, Crenshaw III, Elsholtz HP, He X, Kapiloff MS, Mangalam HJ, Swanson LW, Treacy MN, Rosenfeld MG (1990) A family of POU-domain and Pit-1 tissue-specific transcription factors in pituitary and neuroendocrine development. Annual Reviews Physiology 52: 773–91.

Kelley PM, Harris DJ, Comer BC, Askew JW, Fowler T, Smith SD, Kimberling WJ (1998) Novel mutations in the connexin 26 gene (GJB2) that cause autosomal recessive (DFNB1) hearing loss. American Journal of Human Genetics 62: 792–9.

Kelsell DP, Dunlop J, Stevens HP, Lench NJ, Liang JN, Parry G, Mueller RF, Leigh IM (1997) Connexin 26 mutations in hereditary non-syndromic sensorineural deafness. Nature 387: 80–3.

Khetarpal U (1993) Autosomal dominant sensorineural hearing loss. Further temporal bone findings. Archives of Otolaryngology and Head and Neck Surgery 119: 106–8.

Khetarpal U, Schuknecht HF, Gacek RR, Holmes LB (1991) Autosomal dominant sensorineural hearing loss. Pedigrees, audiologic findings, and temporal bone findings in two kindreds. Archives of Otolaryngology and Head and Neck Surgery 117: 1032–42.

Kubisch C, Schroeder BC, Friedrich T, Lütjohann B, El-Amraoui A, Marlin S, Petit C, Jentsch TJ (1999) KCNQ4, a novel potassium channel expressed in sensory outer hair cells, is mutated in dominant deafness. Cell 96: 437–46.

Li XC, Everett LA, Lalwani AK, Desmukh D, Friedman TB, Green ED, Wilcox ER (1998) A mutation in PDS causes non-syndromic recessive deafness. Nature Genetics 18: 215–17.

Liu XZ, Walsh J, Mburu P, Kendrick-Jones J, Cope MJ, Steel KP, Brown SD (1997a) Mutations in the myosin VIIA gene cause non-syndromic recessive deafness.Nature Genetics 16: 188–90.

Liu XZ, Walsh J, Tamagawa Y, Kitamura K, Nishizawa M, Steel KP, Brown SD (1997b) Autosomal dominant non-syndromic deafness caused by a mutation in the myosin VIIA gene. Nat Genet 17: 268–9.

Lynch ED, Lee MK, Morrow JE, Welcsh PL, Leon PE, King MC (1997) Nonsyndromic deafness DFNA1 associated with mutation of a human homolog of the Drosophila gene diaphanous. Science 278: 1315–18.

Mustapha M, Salem N, Weil D, El-Zir E, Loiselet J, Petit C (1998) Identification of a locus on chromosome 7q31, DFNB14, responsible for prelingual sensorineural non-syndromic deafness. European Journal of Human Genetics 6: 548–51.

Prezant TR, Agapian JV, Bohlman MC, Bu X, Oztas S, Qiu WQ, Arnos KS, Cortopassi GA, Jaber L, Rotter JI, Shohat M, Fischel-Ghodsian N (1993) Mitochondrial ribosomal RNA mutation associated with both antibiotic-induced and non-syndromic deafness. Nature Genetics 4: 289–94.

Probst FJ, Fridell RA, Raphael Y, Saunders TL, Wang AH, Liang Y, Morell RJ, Touchman JW, Lyons RH, Noben-Trauth K, Friedman TB, Camper SA (1998) Correction of deafness in shaker-2 mice by an unconventional myosin in a BAC transgene. Science 280: 1444–7.

Reid FM, Vernham GA, Jacobs HT (1994) A novel mitochondrial point mutation in a maternal pedigree with sensorineural deafness. Human Mutation 3: 243–7.

Richard G, Smith LE, Bailey RA, Itin P, Hohl D, Epstein EH, DiGiovanna JJ, Compton JG, Bale SJ (1998) Mutations in the human connexin gene GJB3 cause erythrokeratodermia variabilis. Nature Genetics 20: 366–9.

Robertson NG, Lu L, Heller S, Merchant SN, Eavey RD, McKenna M, Nadol JB, Miyamoto RT, Linthicum FH, Neto JFL, Hudspeth AJ, Seidman CE, Morton CC, Seidman JG (1998) Mutations in a novel cochlear gene cause DFNA9, a human non-syndromic deafness with vestibular dysfunction. Nature Genetics 20: 299–303.

Rosenfeld MG (1991) POU-domain transcription factors: pou-er-ful developmental regulators. Genes and Development 5: 897–907.

Scott DA, Kraft ML, Stone EM, Sheffield VC, Smith RJH (1998) Connexin mutations and hearing loss. Nature 391: 32.

Scott DA, Wang R, Kreman TM, Sheffield VC, Karnishki LP (1999) The Pendred syndrome gene encodes a chloride-iodide transport protein. Nature Genetics 21: 440–3.

Sevior KB, Hatamochi A, Stewart IA, Bykhovskaya Y, Allen-Powell DR, Fischel-Ghodsian N, Maw MA (1998) Mitochondrial A7445G mutation in two pedigrees with palmoplantar keratoderma and deafness. American Journal of Medical Genetics 75: 179–85.

Thompson DA, Weigel RJ (1998) Characterization of a gene that is inversely correlated with estrogen receptor expression (ICERE-1) in breast carcinomas. European Journal of Biochemistry 252: 169–77.

Usami S, Abe S, Kasai M, Shinkawa H, Moeller B, Kenyon JB, Kimberling WJ (1997) Genetic and clinical features of sensorineural hearing loss associated with the 1555 mitochondrial mutation. Laryngoscope 107: 483–90.

Usami S, Abe S, Weston MD, Shinkawa H, Van Camp G (1999) Non-syndromic hearing loss associated with enlarged vestibular aqueduct is caused by PDS mutations. Human Genetics 104: 188–92.

Vahava O, Morell R, Lynch ED, Weiss S, Kagan ME, Ahituv N, Morrow JE, Lee MK, Skvorak AB, Morton CC, Blumenfeld A, Frydman M, Friedman TB, King MC, Avraham KB (1998) Mutation in transcription factor POU4F3 associated with inherited progressive hearing loss in humans. Science 279: 1950–4.

Van Hauwe P, Everett LA, Coucke P, Scott DA, Kraft ML, Ris-Stalpers C, Bolder CHHM, Otten B, De Vijlder JJM, Dietrich NL, Ramesh A, Srikumari Srisailapathy CR, Parving A, Cremers CWRJ, Willems PJ, Smith RJH, Green ED, Van Camp G (1998) Two frequent missense mutations in Pendred syndrome. Human Molecular Genetics 7: 1099–104.

Van Laer L, Huizing EH, Verstreken M, Van Zuijlen D, Wauters JG, Bossuyt PJ, Van de Heyning P, McGuirt WT, Smith RJH, Willems PJ, Legan PK, Richardson GP, Van Camp G (1998) Nonsyndromic hearing impairment is associated with a mutation in DFNA5. Nature Genetics 20: 194–7.

Verhoeven K, Van Laer L, Kirschhofer K, Legan PK, Hughes DC, Schatteman I, Verstreken M, Van Hauwe P, Coucke P, Chen A, Smith RJH, Somers T, Offeciers FE, Van de Heyning P, Richardson GP, Wachtler F, Kimberling WT, Willems PJ, Govaerts PJ, Van Camp G (1998) Mutations in the human α-tectorin gene cause autosomal dominant non-syndromic hearing impairment. Nature Genetics 19: 60–2.

Wang A, Liang Y, Fridell RA, Probst FJ, Wilcox ER, Touchman JW, Morton CC, Morell RJ, Noben-Trauth K, Camper SA, Friedman TB (1998) Association of unconventional myosin MYO15 mutations with human nonsyndromic deafness DFNB3. Science 280: 1447–51.

Weil D, Blanchard S, Kaplan J, Guilford P, Gibson F, Walsh J, Mburu P, Varela A, Levilliers J, Weston MD, Kelley PM, Kimberling WJ, Wagenaar M, Levi-Acobas F, Larget-Piet D, Munnich A, Steel KP, Brown SDM, Petit C (1995) Defective myosin VIIA gene responsible for Usher syndrome type 1B. Nature 374: 60–1.

Weil D, Kussel P, Blanchard S, Levy G, Levi-Acobas F, Drira M, Ayadi H, Petit C (1997) The autosomal recessive isolated deafness, DFNB2, and the Usher 1B syndrome are allelic defects of the myosin-VIIA gene. Nature Genetics 16: 191–3.

Wenzel K, Manthey D, Willecke K, Grzeschik KH, Traub O (1998) Human gap junction protein connexin31: molecular cloning and expression analysis. Biochemical and Biophysical Research Communications 248: 910–15.

White TW, Deans MR, Kelsell DP, Paul DL (1998) Connexin mutations in deafness. Nature 394: 630–1.

Xia JH, Liu CY, Tang BS, Pan Q, Huang L, Dai HP, Zhang BR, Xie W, Hu DX, Zheng D, Shi XL, Wang DA, Xia K, Yu KP, Liao XD, Feng Y, Yang YF, Xiao JY, Xie DH, Huang JZ (1998) Mutations in the gene encoding gap junction protein beta-3 associated with autosomal dominant hearing impairment. Nature Genetics 20: 370–3.

Yasunaga S, Grati M, Cohen-Salmon M, El-Amraoui A, Mustapha M, Salem N, El-Zir E, Loiselet J, Petit C (1999) A mutation in OTOF, encoding otoferlin, a FER-1-like protein, causes DFNB9, a nonsyndromic form of deafness. Nature Genetics 21: 363–9.

Zelante L, Gasparini P, Estivill X, Melchionda S, D'Agruma L, Govea N, Mila M, Monica MD, Lutfi J, Shohat M, Mansfield E, Delgrosso K, Rappaport E, Surrey S, Fortina P (1997) Connexin26 mutations associated with the most common form of non- syndromic neurosensory autosomal recessive deafness (DFNB1) in Mediterraneans. Human Molecular Genetics 6: 1605–9.

Chapter 19
Connexin 26 (*GJB2*) deafness homepage

(URL:http://www. iro.es./cx26deaf.html editors – X Estivill, P Gasparini, N Lench)

ROBERT MUELLER

Mapping of DFNB1 locus

The first locus for autosomal recessive non-syndromal sensorineural hearing impairment/deafness (ARNSSNHI/D) was assigned to the proximal portion of the long arm of chromosome 13 at 13q11–12 by autozygosity mapping in consanguineous Tunisian families (Guilford et al, 1994). Segregation of polymorphic DNA microsatellites linked to the *DFNB1* locus in familial NSSNBI/D showed that it made an important contribution to ARNSSNHI/D (Maw et al., 1995; Gasparini et al., 1997). An autosomal dominant non-syndromal sensorineural hearing impairment/deafness (ADNSSNHI/D) locus (*DFNA3*) was also mapped to the same region of chromosome 13 (Chaib et al., 1994).

GJB2 mutations cause autosomal recessive and dominant NSSNHI/D

The gene at the *DFNB1* locus was identified in a family in which an inherited disorder of the skin, palmoplantar keratoderma (PPK) and sensorineural hearing impairment/deafness appeared to be inherited as an autosomal dominant disorder linked to polymorphic microsatellite markers at 13q11–q12 (Kelsell et al., 1997). The GJB2 (connexin26) gene, which encodes the gap junction beta-2 protein mapped into this interval, was known to be expressed in the skin making it a positional candidate gene.

176

Analysis of the *GJB2* gene in DNA from people with deafness in the family revealed a T to C missense mutation resulting in the substitution of threonine for methionine (M34T) in the first transmembrane region of the GJB2 protein. A review of the family showed that this mutation appeared to segregate with the hearing impairment/deafness but not the skin disorder. Samples from individuals with ARNSSNHI/D from three complex consanguineous British Pakistani families in which hearing impairment/deafness was known to be linked to the *DFNB1* locus showed affected individuals to be homozygous for two different nonsense mutations of the *GJB2* gene. These two mutations cause premature stop codons in the first and second transmembrane domains of the GJB2 protein, leading to a severely truncated and non-functional GJB2 protein, thus establishing the role of GJB2 in causing ARNSSNHI/D (Kelsell et al., 1997).

Mechanism of Cx26 causing AR and AD NSSNHI/D

The connexins are a large family of proteins widely expressed in different tissues. Six connexin subunits assemble to make a connexon; the association of two connexins between adjacent cells form gap-junctions between cells. Gap junctions are thought to be intercellular communication channels facilitating the passive exchange of ions and small molecules up to one kiloDalton in size between cells. Connexins have highly conserved amino acid sequences and are made up of four transmembrane domains, two extracellular loops, an intracellular loop and a cytoplasmic tail with the amino acid sequence of the loop regions and the length of the cytoplasmic tail distinguishing the different connexins (Kikuchi et al., 1995).

Immunohistochemical studies of the inner ear have shown that GJB2 protein is expressed in the inner ear in the stria vascularis, basement membrane, limbus and spiral prominence of the cochlea (Kelsell et al., 1997). The gap junctions in the cells of the inner ear are thought to be the channels through which potassium ions are recycled from the sensory hair cells through their supporting cells back to the endolymph after the mechanoelectrical transduction of auditory stimuli. Mutations in the *GJB2* gene would lead to loss of function of the GJB2 protein, thus interfering with the recycling of potassium ions.

Mutations in the *GJB2* gene in people with ARNSSNHI/D

After the identification of mutations in the *GJB2* gene in people with ARNSSNHI/D, a number of groups have screened individuals with non-syndromal sensorineural hearing impairment/deafness from a variety of different populations for mutations in the gene. A deletion of a single guanine (G) residue in a stretch of 6 Gs, at nucleotide position 30–35 (also known as 30 or 35delG) was found to account for the majority of *GJB2* mutations (>61%) in families with ARNSSNHI/D (Zelante et al., 1997; Denoyelle et al., 1997; Estivill et al., 1998, Lench et al., 1998). This single base pair deletion alters the reading frame (a frame-shift mutation) generating in a stop codon at codon 13 of the gene, resulting in premature termination of translation leading to a GJB2 protein truncated in the first transmembrane domain. These same studies have shown that in a number of different population groups the majority (up to 80%) of families with ARNSSNHI/D and between one in 10 and one in three sporadically affected individuals with NSSNHI/D occurs due to mutations in the *GJB2* gene.

To date 44 different mutations have been reported in the *GJB2* gene as causing ARNSSNHI/D in a variety of different populations, which include missense, nonsense, deletions, frame-shift and splice site mutations (URL:http://www.iro.es./cx26deaf.html). The majority of mutations reported have been observed only a limited number of times, although the 167delT mutation has been found to be the most common mutation in people of Ashkenazi Jewish origin with ARNSSNHI/D (Kelley et al., 1998; Morrel et al., 1998).

Mutations in the *GJB2* gene in persons with ADNSSNHI/D

The M34T *GJB2* sequence variant reported in the original family segregating PPK and sensorineural hearing impairment/deafness, has also been reported in persons with normal hearing (Kelley et al., 1998). Studies of the frequency of this sequence variant in the general population suggest that it could be a rare polymorphic variant and not be of any functional consequence, although *in vitro* studies in *Xenopus laevis* oocytes of this mutant have shown abnormal channel activity (White et al., 1998). In the family with ADNSSNHI/D, which had mapped the *DFNA3* locus to the same region of chromosome 13, a missense mutation, in which a G is substituted by a cytosine (C), leads to a tryptophan to cysteine substitution at codon 44 (W44C) of *GJB2*, was identified (Denoyelle et al., 1998). This amino acid substitution is located in the first extracellular domain of Cx26 and would interfere with the formation of normal disulphide bonds, which is likely to alter the interaction between connexins of adjacent cells and act in a dominant negative manner.

Genotype-phenotype correlations in NSSNHI/D due to *GJB2* mutations

The hearing impairment in the majority of individuals with ARNSSNHI/D due to a mutation in the *GJB2* gene reported to date is usually prelingual, bilaterally symmetrical with the degree of hearing impairment usually being severe or profound. In a minority, the hearing impairment/deafness is moderate and/or asymmetrical in its severity. There is no apparent correlation of severity of hearing impairment with particular mutations in the *GJB2* gene (Denoyelle et al., 1999). The hearing impairment/deafness in the affected individuals from families with ADNSSNHI/D, although prelingual in onset, was progressive with the high frequencies being more severely affected.

References

Chaib H, Lina-Granade G, Guilford P, Plauchu H, Livilliers J, Morgon A, Petit C (1994) A gene responsible for a dominant form of neurosensory non-syndromic deafness maps to the *NSRD1* recessive deafness gene interval. Human Molecular Genetics 3: 2219–22.

Denoyelle F, Weil D, Maw MA, Wilcox SA, Lench NJ, Allen-Powell DR, Osborn AH, Dahl H-HM, Middleton A, Houseman MJ, Dodé C, Marlin S, Boulila-ElGaïed A, Grati M, Ayadi H, BenArab S, Bitoun P, Lina-Granade G, Godet J, Levilliers J, Garabédian EN, Mueller RF, Gardner RJM, Petit C (1997) Prelingual deafness: high prevalence of a 30delG mutation in the connexin 26 gene. Human Molecular Genetics 6: 2173–7.

Denoyelle F, Lina-Granade G, Plauchu H, Bruzzone R, Chaïb H, Lévi-Acobas F, Weil D, Petit C (1998) Connexin 26 gene linked to a dominant deafness. Nature 393: 319–20.

Denoyelle F, Marlin S, Weil D, Moatti L, Chauvin P, Garabedian EN, Petit C (1999) Clinical features of the prevalent form of childhood deafness, DFNB1, due to a connexin-26 gene defect: implications for genetic counselling. Lancet 353: 1298–303.

Estivill X, Fortina P, Surrey S, Rabionet R, Melchionda S, D'Agruarna L, Mansfield E, Rappaport E, Govea N, Milá M, Zelante L, Gasparini P (1998) Connexin-26 mutations in sporadic and inherited sensorineural deafness. Lancet 351: 394–8.

Gasparini P, Estivill X, Volpini V, Totara A, Castellvi-Bel S, Govea, N, Milá M, Della Monica M, Venruto V, De Benedetto M, Stanziale P, Zelante L, Mansfield ES, Sandkuijl L, Surrey S, Fortina P (1997) Linkage of DFNB1 to non-syndromic neurosensory autosomal-recessive deafness gene interval. European Journal of Human Genetics 5: 83–8.

Guilford, P, Ben Arab S, Blanchard S, Levilliers J, Weissenbach J, Bolkhaia A, Petit A (1994) A non-syndromic form of neurosensory, recessive deafness maps to the pericentromeric region of chromosome 13q. Nature Genetics 6: 24–8.

Kelley PM, Harris DJ, Comer BC, Askew JW, Fowler T, Smith SD, Kimberling WJ (1998) Novel mutations in the connexin 26 (GJB2) that cause autosomal recessive (DFNB1) hearing loss. American Journal of Human Genetics 62: 792–9.

Kelsell DP, Dunlop J, Stevens HP, Lench NJ, Liang JN, Parry G, Mueller RF, Leigh IM (1997) Connexin 26 mutations in hereditary non-syndromic, sensorineural deafness. Nature 387: 80–3.

Kikuchi T, Kimura RS, Paul DL, Adams JC (1995) Gap junctions in the rat cochlea: immunohistochemical and ultrastructural analysis. Anatomy and Embryology 191: 101–18.

Lench NJ, Houseman M, Newton V, Van Camp G, Mueller RF (1998) Connexin-26 mutations in sporadic non-syndromal sensorineural deafness. Lancet 351: 415.

Maw MA, Allen-Powell DR, Goodey RJ, Stewart IA, Nancarrow DJ, Hayward NK, Gardner RJM (1995) The contribution of the DFNB1 locus to neurosensory deafness in a Caucasian population. American Journal of Human Genetics 57: 629–35.

Morrel RJ, Kim HJ, Hood LJ, Goforth L, K Friderici, Fisher R, Van Camp G, Berlin CI, Oddoux C, Ostrer H, Keats B, Friedman TB (1998) Mutations in the connexin 26 gene (GJB2) among Ashkenazi Jews with nonsyndromic recessive deafness. New England Journal of Medicine 339: 1500–5.

White TW, Deans MR, Kelsell DP, Paul DL, (1998) Connexin mutations in deafness. Nature 394: 630–1.

Zelante L, Gasparini P, Estivill X, Melchionda S, D'AGruma L, Govea N, Milá M, Della Monica M, Lutfi J, Shohat M, Mansfield E, Delgrosso K, Rappaport E, Surrey S, Fortina P (1997) Connexin26 mutations, associated with the most common form of non-syndromic autosomal recessive deafness (DFNB1) in Mediterraneans. Human Molecular Genetics 6: 1605–9.

Index